K. Howorka, Functional Insulin Treatment

Springer
Berlin
Heidelberg
New York
Barcelona
Budapest
Hong Kong
London
Milan
Paris
Santa Clara
Singapore
Tokyo

Kinga Howorka

Functional Insulin Treatment

Principles, Teaching Approach and Practice

With Forewords by
M. Berger and J. S. Skyler

2nd Edition

With 31 Figures and 10 Tables

Springer

Kinga Howorka, M.D.
International Study Group on Functional Insulin Treatment
Department of Biomedical Engineering and Physics
University of Vienna, Allgemeines Krankenhaus, Leitstelle 4L
Währinger Gürtel 18–20, A-1090 Wien

Translated by Kathryn Nelson

Adapted from the Fourth German Edition:
Funktionelle Insulintherapie – Lehrinhalte, Praxis und Didaktik
Vierte, überarbeitete Auflage, Springer-Verlag Berlin Heidelberg 1996

ISBN-13: 978-3-540-60352-8 e-ISBN-13: 978-3-642-79997-6
DOI: 10.1007/978-3-642-79997-6

Die Deutsche Bibliothek – CIP-Einheitsaufnahme
Howorka, Kinga: Functional insulin treatment : principles, teaching approach and practice ; with 10 tables / Kinga Howorka. With forewords by M. Berger and J. S. Skyler. [Transl. by Kathryn Nelson]. – 2. ed. –
Berlin ; Heidelberg ; New York ; Barcelona ; Budapest ; Hong Kong ; London ; Milan ; Paris ; Santa Clara ; Singapore ; Tokyo : Springer 1996
Dt. Ausg. u. d. T.: Howorka, Kinga: Funktionelle, nahe-normoglykämische Insulinsubstitution
ISBN-13. 978-3-540-60352-8

Typesetting (media conversion): FotoSatz Pfeifer GmbH, Gräfelfing/München

SPIN: 10515154 23/3134 – 5 4 3 2 1 0 – Printed on acid-free paper

To our insulin-dependent patients who – unable to comply with the demands of conventional insulin treatment – have been instrumental in the development of the concept of functional insulin use.

Foreword

The absence of endogenous insulin secretion is the fundamental defect in Type I diabetes mellitus. Thus, the availability of insulin as a therapeutic agent, commencing in 1922, offered the hope that diabetes could be treated. The introduction of insulin indeed sustained the lives of those afflicted with Type I diabetes. But, the devastating effects of chronic complications often ravaged patients with the disease. Yet, it is abundantly clear that the frequency, severity, and progression of those complications is directly linked to the degree of glycemic control over time. Therefore, it is incumbant upon physicians and patients to develop successful strategies for attaining and maintaining meticulous glycemic control, whilst minimizing the associated risks consequent to hypoglycemia. Not an easy task.

An approach to insulin replacement is to regidly define daily activity (and the requisite energy expenditure), match that with a carefully planned and rigorous meal plan, and define the insulin requirement needed to allow utilization of those calories for that degree of energy expenditure. In theory, if all of these parameters are kept absolutely constant from day to day, glycemia should be predictable and control achievable.

Who amongst us without diabetes follows a rigidly defined program of activity and eating? The fact is that neither we nor our patients are robots capable of reproducibility following the identical daily schedule for years. The issue becomes whether or not a flexible lifestyle can be compatible with meticulous glycemic control.

The answer is *yes*. And, in this cleverly crafted book, Dr. Kinga Howorka defines how it can be done. Dealing with diabetes of her patients, Dr. Howorka has developed a therapeutic strateg which she calls "functional insulin treatment". The strategy fundamentally is one that advocates a flexible life style, in which one tailors the insulin therapy to the life style. Thus, patients take multiple daily insulin injections (or use an insulin pump) and measure their blood glucose several times daily.

The principles used by Dr. Howorka are being more widely accepted amongst diabetes specialists. What she has done, however, is to take these principles to a new higher level of practice, and has developed a scheme to programmatically implement her program of functional insulin treatment. Her detailed description of this program provides a framework by which other physicians can replicate her successes. The method is well worth careful scrutiny by all of us who *care* for and about patients with Type I diabetes.

Miami, Florida
June, 1991

Professor Jay S. Skyler, M.D.
Professor, University of Miami

Foreword to the First German-Language Edition

During the last ten years, clinical diabetology has been set in motion. This new orientation has become especially clear in the care of patients with type I (insulin-dependent) diabetes mellitus. The reasons for this process of rethinking in diabetology are manifold, and by occurring together in time they have mutually amplified each other's effects. The decisive evidence for a causal relationship between hyperglycemia and the development of microangiopathic late complications of diabetes – which leading diabetologists have long postulated and vehemently advocated as being biologically logical – has finally made (near) normoglycemia the generally recognized goal of preventive therapy. The discovery of glycosylated hemoglobin as a long-term parameter of the quality of metabolic control made it possible for the first time to verify whether therapeutic goals were actually being reached. Only then was it possible to aim at metabolic normalization by means of a *rational* therapy based on systematic intervention with verifiable effects. This process of enlightenment allowed the *demystification* of therapeutic goals and methods: Type I diabetes was once more recog nized as a direct consequence of an (almost) complete deficiency of an endocrine hormone – insulin. Insulin *substitution* has finally come to the fore as the crucial cornerstone of treatment.

If insulin treatment is to be a true replacement therapy, then it must imitate physiological insulin secretion. This necessarily entailed the rediscovery of the importance of regular insulin, which during the last 50 years had been almost completely pushed into the background compared with the delayed-acting insulins. On the basis of new knowledge regarding the physiology of insulin secretion in healthy subjects, it made sense to differentiate between basal and prandial insulin requirements for insulin replacement in type I (insulin-dependent) diabetes as well. The replacement of basal and prandial insulin separately from and independently of each other became the hallmark of the so-called intensified insulin therapies. The logical consequences of this were that (1) the success of insulin substitution had to be systematically verified by means of regular blood glucose monitoring. With the help of the self-monitoring methods developed toward the end of the 1970s, this task could be transferred to the patient. (2) In view of the diversity and variability of the factors which influence blood glucose levels in daily life, successful equilibration of glucose metabolism could only be achieved by extensive delegation of rights and responsibilities during treatment to the diabetic patient himself. Patient education, i.e., the motivation and training of the patient for self-therapy, therefore became an essential basis of therapeutic success. (3) Systematic self-monitoring of blood glucose and autonomous adaptation of insulin dose, with the transfer of the corresponding rights and responsibilities to the patient, allowed insulin substitution therapy to approach more and more closely to physiological insulin secretion. Previously common dogmas aimed at the *regulation* of lifestyle and eating behavior could now be abandoned. Rigid rules for carrying out physical activity at exactly the same time each day, regimenting the times for getting up and going to bed, and the exact planning of what was to be eaten and when, could all be discarded. Long before diabetologists had begun to debate the liberalization in the lifestyle of type I diabetes patients, our patients had come to these conclusions and were attempting to put them into practice.

The gains in quality of life and flexibility of lifestyle produced by dropping rules and regulations that had tried – without success – to force the rhythm of daily life as well as eating habits into the straightjacket of a completely unphysiological insulin therapy (e.g., two injections of delayed-acting insulin per day), were bought at the cost of accepting additional duties. The reward was good metabolic control (including the abandoning of the previously frequent hospital stays for the dubious process of readjusting the therapy regime) in spite of a freer way of life.

This new orientation in the therapy of type I (insulin-dependent) diabetes mellitus cannot be solely attributed to the latest scientific and technological developments and discoveries. It also coincides with a particular sociocultural trend of recent years, namely, the dissolution of traditional authoritarian structures. There could be practically no more paternalistic and dependent relationship than that of the traditional relationship of the (chronically ill) type I diabetic patient and his physician. The collapse of this completely inefficient, even inhuman and quite unjustifiable subordination and the emancipation of the patient within a cooperative partnership with the physician represents a prerequisite for the successful performance of intensive insulin therapy by the patient. Parallel social developments in the 1980s have lent support to both physicians and patients during this mutually difficult process of reorientation in their relationship.

In this report of her experiences with functional insulin treatment (FIT), the system of intensified insulin therapy which she has developed, Kinga Howorka has successfully journeyed along the way toward an autonomous insulin substitution therapy for type I diabetic persons as well as toward liberalization of diet and lifestyle. In fact she has traveled further along this path than others have dared to go. While other centers with basically identical philosophies have tried much more gradually to establish self-responsibility and therapeutic flexibility in individual patients, FIT sets out from the principle of a fundamental and far-reaching elevation of the standards for therapy, a priori for any type I diabetic patient who can be motivated to participate. The results are impressive and equally attractive to physicians and patients. The detailed work *with* the patient in the framework of a complex, unusually systematic and intensive training program was the key to this suc cess.

The author has described the theoretical background and practical aspects of this program in extensive detail as a handbook for the cooperation between patient and physician. If readers make the effort to study the text attentively and to apply it with careful evaluation of their own experiences in putting it into practice, then the success of this book will be assured. Great personal commitment, humaneness and cooperative modesty on the part of the physician/diabetes counselor in relation to the patient will, however, be a condition of this success.

The foreword to a manual for a therapeutic method that is still often seen as being somewhat avant-garde would be incomplete if it were not pointed out that the methods of intensified insulin therapy that are currently spreading so successfully, of which this book at present represents the most advanced form, are by no means new. From 1929 until his death, the German pediatrician Karl Stolte (1881–1951) developed and successfully applied an extremely clear and concise scheme for intensified insulin therapy. His therapeutic plan was based on three or more daily injections of regular insulin before the main meals. His patients self-monitored urine glucose before each meal and autonomously varied insulin dose according to the results and the amount of carbohydrates they planned to eat. Delayed-acting insulins and the necessity for sugar substitutes were strictly rejected; dietary prescriptions were liberalized to the extent of a "free" diet with a high component of carbohydrates and restriction of fats, with strict attention being paid to achieving normal metabolic conditions in order to avoid late complications (or as Stolte called them, "after-diseases" of the eyes and kidneys). The main principle of Stolte's teachings was to educate the patient to take responsibility for his own therapy, to be able to act independently of doctors and hospitals. This was based on systematic and intensive training of the diabetic patient in self-monitoring and autonomous adaptation of insulin dose (i. e., insulin substitution in imitation of physiological events, while doing away to a great extent with dietary prescriptions as long as there was freedom from glucosuria). For the lucidity of his writings, Stolte must be regarded as *the* pioneer of modern diabetology. Unfortun ately, he was not able to prevail against the established opinions of the day or against their protagonists. He was misunderstood – either consciously or unconsciously – and was pushed more and more into the role of an outsider.

Due to the reasons previously mentioned, the chances for the ultimate breakthrough of a rational therapy of type I diabetes mellitus, as represented by intensified insulin therapies, particularly FIT, are certainly better *today*. For the good of our patients, we should all take advantage of them.

Düsseldorf,
August, 1986

Professor Michael Berger, M. D.
Department of Metabolism and Nutrition
University of Düsseldorf
WHO Collaborating Center for Diabetes

Author's Preface to the 2nd English Edition

So this is heaven, he thought, and he had to smile at himself (...). In the days that followed, Jonathan saw that there was as much to learn about flight in this place as there had been in life behind him. But with a difference. Here were gulls who thought as he thought. For each of them, the most important thing in living was to reach out and touch perfection in that which they most loved to do, and that was to fly. They were magnificant birds, all of them (...).

Jonathan Livingston Seagull
Richard D. Bach

It has now been finally established that good glycemic control helps to prevent or to stabilize the late complications of diabetes. Quality assurance has now become obligatory in the field of diabetes care. Patient education is commonplace in most diabetes centers and I am led to hope that my cynical comments in the "Intermezzi" in this book are (or soon will be) no longer relevant to the diabetic patient's experience.

In many centers, perhaps especially in the German-speaking world, there is still some confusion concerning terminology for the different forms of insulin treatment. When one thinks of "intensified insulin treatment," the image is generally of something far more onerous and demanding than "conventional" insulin treatment. I am convinced, however, that the type of insulin treatment proposed in this book, the flexible, "functional insulin treatment" (FIT), actually makes life easier and more pleasant for the diabetic patient in the long run. I have been confirmed in this belief by enthusiastic reports from many patients who have gone through the FIT training program. Therefore, I would like to propose a modification of the terminology (Sect. 3.4.), and I would like to thank all those people who have contributed to the clarification of this situation.

Our original program was developed for type I diabetic patients and was entitled "functional insulin substitution." Since many type II diabetic patients also want to learn how to specifically lower their blood sugar and to free themselves of the tyranny of having to eat on schedule, out of "functional insulin substitution" the idea of "functional insulin treatment" has grown. This concept is basically suitable for any *interested* person who injects insulin. Therefore, a new chapter about "FIT" for type II diabetic patients has been included in this edition.

I would like to say a sincere thank-you for all of the criticisms and suggestions which have led to the further improvement, simplification and enrichment of FIT. Only through feedback that includes both enthusiasm for the good parts and rejection of the bad has the development of this concept of *outpatient* diabetes care been made possible.

Many sincere thanks, therefore,
for both.

Kinga Howorka, June 1995

Contents

Both the author and the translator of this book are women and dedicated to the furtherance of feminine causes. Nevertheless, solely in the interests of simplicity, we have kept to traditional use of the pronoun *he* in the examples cited in the text.

1 Introduction

The increasingly widespread availability of systematic, structured diabetes education programs as well as self-monitoring techniques and the use of improved methods of insulin administration have brought about decisive progress in the therapy of type I (insulin-dependent) diabetes in recent years. Chronic hyperglycemia is nonetheless still present in the vast majority of type I diabetic patients. One reason for this poor therapeutic success is the fact that patient education remains inadequate (Mühlhauser et al. 1982), especially in the face of the need to consider fluctuations in individual insulin requirements (Bruns et al. 1983) and variations in insulin absorption kinetics (Berger et al. 1982). Unfortunately, the failure of therapy is often simply blamed on a lack of patient motivation and cooperation.

The necessity for changing the traditional concept of type I diabetes treatment arises from the recognition of the root cause of the failure of conventional insulin therapy. For over 60 years, since the discovery and first use of insulin for treating type I diabetes, it has been assumed that the insulin-dependent patient should, can, and is willing to adapt his life to the action of the insulin he injects. This well-known premise of insulin therapy has been shown to be false in the majority of cases. **Most type I diabetic patients cannot and will not adapt their lifestyles to accommodate the activity of their insulin.**

In 1983 Berger et al. wrote in their book on the practice of insulin therapy, "The main goal of insulin therapy is to achieve normoglycemia in order to prevent late complications, while at the same time maintaining the greatest possible flexibility in the lifestyle of the patient. This is only feasible when the patient himself learns as far as possible to carry out adaptations in his medication." The concept of functional insulin treatment (FIT) represents a further development of this line of thought. The essence of FIT is to imitate physiological conditions as closely as possible by differentiated insulin administration according to function (fulfilling basal requirements, compensating for food intake, or correcting blood glucose excursions caused by other factors).

Our group set the following goals:

1. To define the minimum conditions under which an adult with type 1 diabetes can functionally use insulin, while simultaneously maintaining near-normoglycemia inspite of flexibility in food intake;
2. To develop a method for determining rules (i.e., algorithms) for the functional use of insulin; and
3. To work out a teaching approach for the transmission of FIT to patients in other centers.

Whether we have achieved these goals can be judged at least partly by the fact that the German editions of both the present book for physicians and diabetes educators and the accompanying handbook for lay persons (K. Howorka: Insulin-dependent? The functional use of insulin. Patient's handbook. Kirchheim Publishers, Mainz, 5th edition 1995), were already sold out within a few months after publication. These two books are intended to complement each other in a multilevel teaching plan. The present book defines the principles of functional insulin treatment and describes the contents, media and techniques of a patient training program. The accompanying handbook contains explicit instructions for patients.

FIT has the following goals:

1. Relative normoglycemia with nearly normal hemoglobin A1c and no severe hypoglycemia.
2. Far-reaching flexibility in food intake and lifestyle, i.e., the insulin-dependent diabetic person should be practically able to live like a nondiabetic.
3. These goals should be attainable with an "acceptable" degree of exertion, which we arbitrarily define as about 10 minutes of time and a few (10–12) "painful seconds" per day. This effortresults primarily from self-monitoring, especially since attempts to substitute for a blood glucose sensor are still not very satisfactory. Should this exertion seem too great to you or your patients, it can be decreased somewhat, but only at the cost of one of the first two goals: either at the cost of normoglycemia or of a flexible lifestyle.

There is currently only one strategy available that can hope to fulfill patient wishes for normoglycemia, a normal lifestyle and simplicity of therapeutic measures. Only the **separate subst itution of basal and prandial insulin secretion, independently of each other**, allows sufficient predictability of blood glucose dynamics after administration of insulin or carbohydrates. The **imitation of the beta cell's blood glucose sensor** is decisive for the effectiveness of insulin substitution. At present this is only possible by measuring blood glucose several times a day and **immediately correcting** deviations from the desired goal.

The strategy of functional insulin treatment is based on active and self-responsible participation by the patient, who must be **capable and willing** to self-monitor his blood glucose, estim ate his dietary intake and insulin requirements and choose his insulin dose accordingly.

The method of insulin administration is contingent on the necessary separation of fasting and meal-related insulins, which must be substituted independently of each other. The FIT strategy is therefore possible either with controlled insulin infusion (for reasons of practicability, simplest with continuous, subcutaneous insulin infusion, CSII), or with multiple daily injections of regular (soluble) and delayed-acting insulin. Twice daily injections of delayed-acting insulin have proven satisfactory in achieving a level of basal insulin equivalent to that with continuous insulin infusion. The comparability of these procedures has been repeatedly demonstrated (Rizza et al. 1980; Reeves et al. 1982; Schiffrin et al. 1982). The decision as to whether multiple daily injections or CSII should be used can be left safely to the patient.

FIT can be seen as a continuing further development of earlier types of insulin therapy. There are some characteristics, however, which enable one to distinguish whether true functional insulin treatment is being carried out. For example, one needs only to ask an insulin-dependent patient, "What do you inject?" This usually means what kind of insulin, how much, and what diet has been prescribed. If the patient answers without hesitation, "X units of this insulin plus Y units of that insulin in the morning and X units of this plus Z units of that in the evening," one can be sure that it is not FIT. A patient who is using FIT cannot answer this question so easily. He would probably answer, "It depends." Simply expressed, it depends on what he eats and how high his blood sugar level is. Since insulin administration under FIT is a function of need, the FIT patient might say, "When I fast, I inject X units of long-acting insulin, when I eat, I inject enough regular insulin to cover the amount of carbohydrates in the meal, and when my blood sugar goes above a certain level, I inject an extra dose of regular insulin to lower it again."

This book came into being in order to create a common basis for communication between therapists (physicians, nurses, dietitians, diabetes educators) and patients. Its purpose is to help therapists to counsel patients in carrying out functional insulin treatment. In the interests of patients, it is important for diabetes educators, nurses, dietitians and physicians to maintain a uniform counseling policy. I am conscious of the fact that the strategies presented here, which are based on experiences at our center and at other diabetes centers using FIT, can be neither complete nor final, even though they result from work with thousands of patients. If you should feel certain information is missing from this book, if you disagree or if you have found better solutions to the same problems, I would be grateful if you would let me know. Any new experiences or ideas which would contribute to improving these methods are very important.

The information contained in the many existing textbooks on insulin treatment will not be repeated here. The contribution of this book lies rather in outlining the practical, didactic, psychological and content-related consequences of FIT within the framework of the education and counseling of type I diabetic persons. The goal of previous diabetes education programs has been to adapt the patient to the conditions of the therapy. **The goal of FIT is to adapt the therapy to the life circumstances of the patient.**

Naturally not all of the contents of this book are new. The essential importance of patient education in the self-treatment of diabetes mellitus has often been pointed out, among others by Joslin (1924), Assal et al. (1982) and Berger (1983b). A number of approaches have already been made to a more physiological, function-related use of insulin (Skyler et al. 1979, Turner et al. 1982). Decisive progress in the development of functional insulin treatment only became possible in the 1980s, however, when self-monitoring of blood glucose began to be widely used (Schiffrin et al. 1982a, 1983; Mühlhauser et al. 1984). Through the reintroduction of regular insulin and multiple daily injections, insulin dosage has become more and more contingent on glycemic level (Skyler et al. 1981; Bernstein 1981). Portable insulin pumps and continuous subcutaneous insulin infusion have also created conditions conducive to the development of functional insulin treatment (Skyler et al. 1982; Sonnenberg, 1983). The results of investigations on the insulin production of healthy persons (Waldhäusl et al. 1979) have added further knowledge. Since FIT is based on the active participation of the patient, insights on coping with a chronic disease from motivational psychology (Gfeller and Assal 1979) and transactional analysis (Berne 1961; Harris 1967, 1985) as well as model-building with the help of neurolinguistic programming (Grinder and Bandler 1976) or solution focus (de Shazer 1988), are extremely important. But the final impulse for developing – and above all, for disseminating – these methods was given by the wishes and experiences of the patients themselves. In a way this book is a collection of tested recipes for changing a "life adapted to the action profile of insulin" into a "life with adapted insulin use." Many aspects of FIT simply grew out of daily experience.

I have been able to gather a number of experiences with various methods of patient education through visits to leading diabetes (education) centers (among others, the International Diabetes Center in Minneapolis, 1984: Donnell Etzwiler; the University of Miami, 1984: Jay Skyler; the University Medical Clinic in Düsseldorf, 1985: Michael Berger; Hvidore Hospital in Copenhagen, 1985: Claus Kühl; Toronto General Hospital, 1985: Bernard Zinman; Children's Hospital in Montreal, 1985: Alicia Schiffrin; the Joslin Clinic in Boston, 1985: Leo Krall; the New York Diabetes Center in Mamaroneck, 1985: Richard Bernstein; Grady Memorial Hospital in Atlanta, 1987: John Davidson). I am especially grateful for the hours and, indeed, days and nights of discussion and the extraordinary helpfulness that was shown me.

The unsatisfactory results of conventional treatment methods in type I diabetes have been repeatedly shown (Czerwenka-Howorka et al. 1984c; Waldhäusl et al. 1985). Considering the current status of insulin therapy, it is understandable that over 95% of our informed patients have decided that FIT with multiple daily injections or CSII is the only practicable and reasonable treatment alternative. But until the termination of the DCCT, many physicians and diabetes counselors were skeptical, believing that the majority of patients would not accept FIT because "so many insulin injections are too painful ... it is too difficult to predict blood glucose dynamics after insulin administration or carbohydrate intake ... the patient might become overly preoccupied with the disease due to the constant blood glucose measurements ... 4–5 blood sugar measurements per day are too many to expect ... self-monitoring might make the patient neurotic ... pumps are really too dangerous ... the methods are still not developed enough ... there is still too little scientific support ... it's too complicated ... there is too great a danger of hypoglycemia, which would be bad for the eyes ... it's too early for this patient, or too late for that one ... it could cause weight gain ... the patients would eat nothing but chocolate ... they would con tinually overinsulinize themselves ... they would make a mess of things ... this type of thing has been tried before and didn't work ... injecting regular insulin is old hat ... it's still too new ... it would be too expensive in the long run ... it only works well at the beginning, while motivation is still high ... there are so many different opinions in diabetology ... one simply can't allow patients to do it ... FIT would only work with highly intelligent (motivated, self-responsible etc.) patients ... because ..."

Should you still agree with the majority of these opinions and doubts, then it would be advisable to read (perhaps exclusively) the sections that begin with the title "Intermezzo." There, evidence has been gathered and ways suggested to confirm these opinions and to convince oneself that FIT is not possible after all.

If, however, you should wish to counsel patients successfully, or if you are simply one of those diabetologists who cannot tolerate it when patients are better informed than they themselves, then you should also read the other chapters. For this book was written with the conviction that without cooperation and partnership between the diabetes counselor and the patient, the self-treatment of insulin-dependent diabetes (which is probably the only efficient treatment currently available) could not be carried out successfully.

In conclusion, a few remarks on the confusion which presently reigns regarding the nomenclature of various forms of insulin therapy. The basis for the developments of the last few years was the introduction of "intensified" insulin therapy, founded on the cooperation of the patient and the availability of self-monitoring of blood glucose. The term "intensified" is not necessarily correct for functional insulin treatment, however, since the total effort involved is much smaller once a patient has been trained in FIT than it is for the usual forms of "intensified" insulin therapy (which generally involve 2–3 injections daily plus extensive efforts to achieve a regular diet). Moreover, the concept of "intensified" insulin therapy is also used differently by different centers. We will go into more detail regarding the overlapping of various therapeutic concepts and difficulties with nomenclature in Sect. 3.4, "Strategies of insulin treatment."

The name we originally gave to our program, "NIS," which was derived in 1983 from "near-normoglycemic insulin substitution," is not 100% accurate for describing functional insulin treatment, since it only describes the goal, not the method. We decided to keep the name "NIS" for the first three German editions of this book because it was already familiar to many, but we feel that "FIT" is more appropriate. The concepts "functional insulin treatment" ("FIT") and "functional, near-normoglycemic insulin substitution" ("NIS") are used synonymously at present. They refer to the **differentiated use of insulin (administered by means of syringe, pump or insulin pen) according to its function, either for covering basal needs, or food intake, or for correction of hyperglycemia, on the basis of individualized rules or algorithms (with the purpose of achieving near-normoglycemia while maintaining flexibility of lifestyle).**

The use of functional insulin treatment has grown exponentially within the last few years. This trend will probably continue in the coming years (or even decades). The development of rapid acting insulin analogs which work faster than regular insulin will probably also contribute to more "physiological" treatment regimens. If medical and technological progress succeeds in making the jump to closed-loop systems of insulin administration, or if efficient immune intervention or transplantation become feasible, FIT may turn into an automatic normoglycemic insulin substitution, independent of patient cooperation. In the meantime, however, what should we do with insulin requiring diabetes **here and now**?

2 Overview of the Phases of Rehabilitation in Persons with Type I (Insulin-Dependent) Diabetes

FIT is based on the ability of the patient to adapt his actions to a given situation. This requires both appropriate information and sustained motivation.

Our experience during the last few years (with approx. 6000 patient years under FIT) has led us to regard the treatment of type I (insulin-independent) diabetic patients as a rehabilitation process and to divide it into four phases, each containing certain educational modules. We differentiate the following phases:

- **Phase 0:** Preliminary information, initial motivation of the patient
- **Phase I:** Basic diabetes education program with the goal of rational self-adaptation of insulin therapy
- **Phase II:** Training in functional insulin treatment, self-adaptation of insulin dosage – both primary adaptation (for acute blood sugar correction) and secondary adaptation (for algorithm correction)
- **Phase III:** Supervision of self-treatment, regular "updates" of practical and theoretical knowledge, detection and, if necessary, treatment of late complications

All four phases can be carried out on an *outpatient* basis and can be separated from each other in time. Phase 0 and phase III are by nature more suited to individual counseling session s, while phase I (basic diabetes education) and phase II (training in FIT) can be carried out to a large extent in groups. Originally phase II was always carried out immediately after phase I, and the two together were referred to as the FIT (formerly NIS, i.e., near-normoglycemic insulin substitution) program. However, we have found it to be advantageous to both trainers and trainees for the individual phases to be carried out at different times (Fig. 2.1).

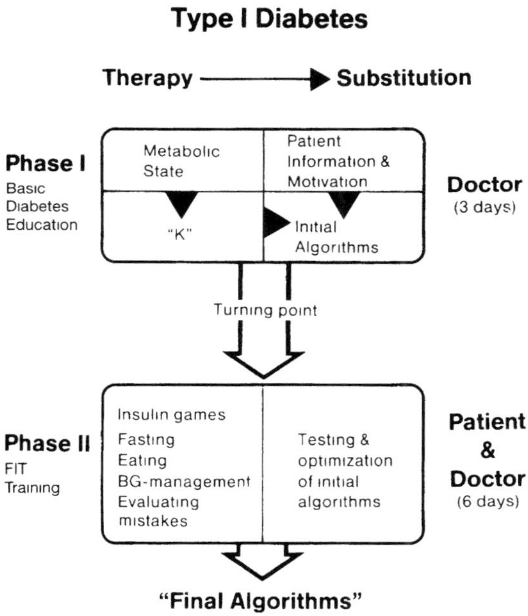

Fig. 2.1. Teaching process for introducing functional insulin treatment: Overview of the FIT program. These phases can be separated and carried out at different times.

An overview of the contents, goals and methods of the four rehabilitation phases is given in Table 2.1. In our experience, an optimal rehabilitation program for type I diabetic patients (achieving individually optimized metabolic control with minimum effort and maximum quality of life) requires a time investment of approx. 40–60 hours.

About 60–90% of this should be in a group teaching format with practical exercises. Due to the amount of training that is necessary, it would be difficult to achieve optimal rehabilitation of type I diabetes without group sessions led by a team of diabetes educators, at least during phases I and II. Unfortunately, this investment is still regarded by many health and pension insurance agencies as too high, so that it is still very difficult to establish the necessary infrastructure and financial support for such a rehabilitation program. Since there is evidence that the methods described here could completely eliminate

Table 2.1. Phases of rehabilitation process for insulin-treated diabetic patients. Modular system of patient education.

	Phase 0 **Preliminary information and motivation**	**Phase I:** **Basic diabetes education**	**Phase II:** **Training in functional insulin treatment**	**Phase III:** **Supervision and update; Rehabilitation in case of associated diseases**	
Module:	• Initial conversation (with physician/counselor) • Exchange of experiences with other diabetics	• Classic diabetes education in group sessions • Events organized by selfhelp groups	• Setting up initial algorithms • Testing and adapting initial algorithms ("insulin games") • Theory and practical consequences	• Supervision (outpatient visits) • FIT Update: Refresher and update group discussion sessions (lasting several hours)	**As needed:** Programs for • Hypertension/ Nephropathy • Hypoglycemia unawareness • Pregnancy and delivery • Weight reduction • Visual handicap
Major goals:	• Initial information and motivation • Determination of quality of metabolic control and late complications • Introduction of multicomponent ("split and mixed regular and NPH or lente") insulin therapy (without premixed insulin) • Provisional setting of therapy goals	• Detailed definition of individual therapy goal (personal decision as to treatment strategy) • Basic information and practical experience	• Learning primary (blood glucose correction) and secondary (algorithm correction) adaptation of insulin dose • Finding out how to achieve optimal quality of life and discovering the limits of functional insulin substitution	• Maintenance of optimal level of knowledge, quality of metabolic control and quality of life • Remotivation • Detection and treatment of late complications and associated diseases	

Table 2.1. (continuation)

	Phase 0 Preliminary information and motivation	Phase I: Basic diabetes education	Phase II: Training in functional insulin treatment	Phase III: Supervision and update; Rehabilitation in case of associated diseases	
Content:	• Possibilities in rehabilitation of IDDM • Literature references • Practical aspects of treatment (Injection technique, selfmonitoring) • Principles of self-variation of insulin dose (Regular and delayed insulins) • Record keeping and evaluation • Hypoglycemia, glucagon • Contact with self-help groups	• Practical consequences of material covered in Phase 0 • Pathophysiology of diabetes • Diet • Insulin-increasing and reducing dosage, multicomponent insulin systems, self-adaptation of dosage • Characteristics, advantages and disadvantages of various treatment strategies ("intensified" vs. "functional" insulin treatment) • Self-monitoring of metabolic control • Hypoglycemia • Late complications of diabetes	• Functional use of insulin (algorithms) • Uniting theory and practice – "Insulin games": short-term tests of FIT-algorithms ("Fasting," "Yielding to Temptation," "Kidney Threshold") • Everyday criteria for evaluating basal and prandial insulin • Primary and secondary dose adaptation • Late complications of diabetes • Special situations	• Detection/removal of individual deficits (theory & practice) • Update of theory and practice • Detection and treatment of late complications of diabetes • Contact with self-help organizations **As needed:** • Program against hypoglycemia unawareness (p. 105) • Pregnancy and delivery preparation (p. 138) • Slimming course (p. 147)	**As needed:** • Hypertension program for elevated BP or microalbuminuria (p. 171): Self-monitoring and control of blood pressure, medications and other measures • Training for visually handicapped: low vision training, mobility training, communication training, training in practical aspects of living • Predialysis counseling if creatinine > 3 mg/dl, contact with nephrologist

Table 2.1. (continuation)

	Phase 0 Preliminary information and motivation	Phase I: Basic diabetes education	Phase II: Training in functional insulin treatment	Phase III: Supervision and update; Rehabilitation in case of associated diseases
Methods:	• Mainly individual counseling • Case history (including previous hospitalizations, attendance at diabetes education programs, hypoglycemic attacks with unconsciousness) • Preliminary clinical examinations	• Group teaching • Teaching conversation • Discussion • Group discussion of insulin dosage using overhead projector for patient records	• Group teaching; Teaching conversation • "Insulin games": "Fasting" (one day); "Yielding to Temptation" (learning to cope with previously "forbidden" foods); "Kidney Threshold" (testing correcting algorithms) • Theoretical material discussed in form of individually adapted "special situations" (pregnancy, sports, surgery, severe hypoglycemia, etc.) • Group discussion of insulin dosage using overhead projector	• Outpatient visits: individual counseling • Structured group teaching programs: teaching conversation – Hypertension/Nephropathy – Hypoglycemia prevention group – Pregnancy and delivery preparation – Slimming course • Rehabilitation of visually handicapped: mainly 1:1 training (special trainer) • Counseling for other late complications: individual sessions • FIT-Update: plenary lectures (for up to 100 patients) and discussion in small groups

Table 2.1. (continuation)

	Phase 0 **Preliminary information and motivation**	**Phase I:** **Basic diabetes education**	**Phase II:** **Training in functional insulin treatment**	**Phase III:** **Supervision and update; Rehabilitation in case of associated diseases**
Dimension	1–3 hours (1–2 sessions)	10–18 hours	16–30 hours	**Proportion of group teaching/Dimension:** • Supervision: 0.5–1 hour/3 months (individual outpatient visits) • FIT-Update: 2-day group program (approx. 14 h/year); cooperation with self-help organizations, exchanging experiences, etc. • Hypertension program: group teaching, 3 sessions, approx. 5 hours each • Training for visually handicapped: individual training, 5–150 hours (mobility training for the blind = 50–70 hours) • Hypoglycemia prevention program: 2 sessions a 5 hours + individual work • Pregnancy preparation: 1 day • Slimming course: 8 sessions approx. 3 hours each
Proportion led by diabetes counselor (%):	50–75%	50–90%	50–80%	
Proportion of group counseling/ group teaching	Generally low, can be up to 50%	75–100%	75–90%	
Proportion of practical exercises	Approx. 30%	30–50%	40–60%	

hospitalizations for modifying insulin treatment (see Chap. 16, "Overview of experience and results"), this is ultimately not a rational attitude. It is to be hoped that more farsighted judgment will prevail in the future.

We believe that each phase of this rehabilitation program is important. It would be a mistake to omit any one phase, since each has a different, but equally important goal.

Phase 0 is decisive for the motivation of the patient and for building up a positive relationship between the patient and the physician/diabetes education team. Even patients with a long duration of diabetes should be able to discover new and important information in this phase.

The emphasis during phase 0 is on motivating the patient for self-care and self-variation of insulin dose on the basis of self-monitoring. To do this it is necessary to introduce the basics of blood glucose and urine glucose testing. It is also helpful to point out literature that he should read before beginning phase I. For patients on two injections of mixed insulin per day, it has proven useful to switch to separate injections of regular (soluble) and delayed-acting insulin both mornings and evenings immediately, even on the first day of counseling. This creates a four-component regimen consisting of "split and mixed regular plus NPH or lente insulin" (Skyler 1981), which the patient can more easily adapt to his daily routine. Self-variation of insulin dose must, of course, be based on good record-keeping, and at this stage it is worthwhile to use one of the conventional diaries for diabetic patients.

When a patient has learned to self-monitor his glycemic state regularly, is able to make some independent variations in his insulin dose, and shows interest in learning more, then he is registered for **phase I**, which is a standard diabetes education program (Muehlhauser et al. 1982). In this phase patients are given extensive information about the nature of their disease and about the current state of knowledge concerning possible forms of treatment. The various strategies for insulin treatment (conventional and intensified insulin therapy, functional insulin treatment), and also various means of insulin delivery (continuous insulin infusion, conventional syringes, insulin pens, etc.) are compared with each other and the advantages and disadvantages are discussed. Considerable motivation for switching to FIT arises from the prospect of attaining normoglycemia with a flexible diet. Even patients who are afraid of multiple daily injections or an insulin pump usually are willing to give FIT at least a short trial. Afterwards, almost no one decides to go back to conventional therapy with one or two injections per day.

The patient's total daily insulin requirement can be estimated on the basis of the previous insulin dose and the glycemic level attained under it, taking the patient's diet, amount of physical activity and whether there was glucosuria or ketonuria into consideration. Comparison with the theoretical insulin requirement, which can be calculated from the insulin production of healthy subjects (Waldhäusl et al. 1979), gives a measure of current (global or average) insulin sensitivity (expressed as the quotient K; see Sect. 4.1, "Initial algorithms") for the individual patient. The K quotient aids in setting up approximate initial **algorithms (or rules)** for determining insulin dosage, thus giving the patient a provisional answer to the following questions:

- "How high is my fasting insulin requirement?"
- "How high is my meal-related insulin requirement?" (i.e., "How much insulin do I need for a specified amount of carbohydrates?")
- "How can I correct my current level of blood glucose (either with insulin or carbohydrates), if it deviates from my target level?"

Only after finding a provisional answer to these questions, i.e., only after setting up a working hypothesis for formulating the insulin dosage algorithms, can **phase II** of the rehabilitation process begin. This involves an abrupt change in treatment strategy. Instead of the previous conventional therapy, in which the patient plays a passive-receptive role, simply administering the insulin dosage prescribed by his doctor and eating a prescribed amount of carbohydrates at set times in order to prevent hypoglycemia, he now actively takes over responsibility for his treatment. *The clear-cut algorithms or rules for insulin application enable the patient to make independent decisions as to insulin dosage and food intake and to assume responsibility for his blood sugar level at any given time.*

The transfer of this responsibility from the doctor to the patient occurs abruptly, not least for psychodynamic reasons. This step, which can occur several weeks or even months after completion of the basic diabetes education program, is the true beginning of FIT, i.e., the actual training in the functional use of insulin.

After the switch to FIT, phase II includes the application and, if necessary, optimization of the initial algorithms by the patient himself

Table 2.2. Suggested schedule for FIT teaching program (phase I and phase II of the rehabilitation process).
The time required for each individual teaching unit is approx. 3–4 hours. Group discussions of current self-monitoring records should be held daily. In order to facilitate evaluation and discussion during the training program, individual self-monitoring records should be written onto transparencies and projected with an overhead projector.

Basic Diabetes Education: Phase I

Unit I:
- Wishes and goals.
- Self-monitoring I: Self-monitoring of blood glucose; techniques of drawing blood (with and without finger-pricking devices); glucose meters; visual evaluation of test strips; parallel measurements; other parameters (urine glucose, acetone, HbA_{1c}, MBG); keeping self-monitoring records (use of transparencies for discussion during training program). Knowledge test 1.
- Function of insulin; insulin deficiency; types of diabetes; late complications; goals of diabetes therapy; basic principles of self-variation of insulin dose.
- Diet I: Calculation of carbohydrates; record-keeping and analysis.

Unit II:
- Insulin in healthy persons I; self-monitoring II.
- Strategies of insulin treatment; types of insulin; history of insulin therapy from the viewpoint of the diabetic patient.
- Acute complications (outline); hypoglycemia; glucagon; discussion of self-monitoring records; self-variation of insulin dose; discussion. DKA.
- Diabetes inheritance. Pregnancy.

Unit III:
- Self-monitoring in practice: Urine glucose; acetone; discussion of self-monitoring records; HbA_{1c}.
- Diet II: Practical aspects.
- Insulin in healthy persons II.
- Insulin treatment (contin.); technical developments in insulin administration; practical aspects of insulin infusion pumps; insulin pens, etc.
- Late complications of diabetes

Unit IV:
- Diet III: Energy content of food; prandial (meal-related) insulin requirements. Glycemic index.
- Practice of intensified insulin therapy.
- Vacations and travel.
- Interpretation of metabolic parameters; algorithms for functional insulin treatment, practice in calculating current insulin deficit and preparation for switch to FIT (optional).
- Discussion of self-monitoring records; general discussion and critique of procedures. Knowledge test 2.

Turning point:
Therapy modification to FIT

Training in FIT: Phase II

Unit I:
- Algorithms for functional insulin use; practice in calculation of insulin deficit; switch to FIT; group discussion of self-monitoring records.
- Routine criteria and simple tests for evaluating FIT algorithms; description of "insulin games."
- Problems in use of regular insulin; kinetics of insulin action.
- Instructions for the insulin game, "Yielding to Temptation"; assembly of a FIT "minikit."

Unit II:
- Group discussion of self-monitoring records and results of (optional) "Yielding to Temptation."
- Summary of routine criteria and tests for algorithm evaluation; secondary adjustment of algorithms.
- Modification of kinetics: Altering the of rate of absorption of carbohydrates and insulin.
- Hypoglycemia: Classification; causes; prevention; therapy; glucagon.
- The dawn phenomenon and its consequences for basal insulin (outline). Discussion of contingency plans for hypothetical problem situations.
- Instructions for the fasting exercise.

Unit III:
Fasting exercise
- Discussion of fasting exercise; interpretation of self-monitoring records.
- Basal insulin substitution (adjustment of the basal rate).
- Costs of diabetes treatment; insurance; late complications; limits of substitution.
- Insulin substitution in special situations I: Physical activity and other situations with a reduction in insulin requirement; principles of primary and secondary adjustment of insulin dosage.
- Discussion of procedures for determining kidney threshold: Definition of basal conditions; checking correction algorithms; raising and lowering blood glucose; threshold determination.

Unit IV:
- Determination of kidney threshold; discussion of results.
- Discussion of secondary adjustment of algorithms.
- Insulin substitution in special situations II: Increases in insulin requirement.
- Summary of the most important rules for FIT: Secondary adjustment – rules for algorithm modification.

Unit V:
- Discussion of self-monitoring records.
- Insulin substitution in special situations III: Miscellaneous.
- Late complications: Reasons for checkups.
- Pregnancy; contraception; heredity.
- Summary: Routine criteria for evaluating FIT algorithms. Knowledge test 3.

Unit VI:
- Medical reports; appointments for checkups; prescriptions; diabetes I. D.; equipment check (insulin, test strips, glucagon, etc.).
- General discussion and critique; open questions; concluding remarks.

under the physician's constant supervision. In this phase the everyday problems involved in dosing insulin according to function are discussed using real-life examples of problem situations. The most important goal of the FIT program is for the patient to acquire the skills necessary for judging the efficacy of his insulin substitution, so that he can correct his blood sugar whenever necessary (primary adjustment of insulin dosage), and independently make necessary adaptations in the algorithms (i.e., secondary adjustment) to accommodate any changes that may occur in the conditions of insulin sensitivity. (See Chap. 8, "Rules for modification of algorithms".)

It is extremely important to realize that even after the completion of phase II, i.e., after mastering functional insulin treatment, the process of rehabilitation is not over. Now **phase III** of the rehabilitation process begins, in which there is a new doctor/patient relationship. The doctor becomes a counselor and supervisor – to be contacted as needed – who is responsible for updating the patient's practical and theoretical knowledge.

In view of the fact that late complications may already be present, it must not be forgotten that normoglycemia alone is not the solution to all the diabetic patient's problems. For example, antihypertensive treatment should have high priority for all patients with relevant microangiopathy (increased microproteinuria) and/or hypertension. An excellent model of antihypertensive group education for diabetic patients, developed by Mühlhauser et al. (1986), is being increasingly used.

Not even the best rehabilitation and patient education programs will (in the foreseeable future) be able to prevent blindness in diabetic persons who already have severe damage. Thus, it is high time that diabetologists gain the necessary knowledge to aid rehabilitation of patients with visual handicaps or blindness. Such patients and others with severe complications (e.g., patients awaiting or undergoing dialysis) should certainly not be crossed off the list of "interesting cases." Rather they deserve every effort to achieve an optimum rehabilitation. An ideal process of rehabilitation might easily be tailored using various optional structured group teaching programs (as hypoglycemia prevention, slimming course ...).

A number of purely pedagogical suggestions for organizing and presenting the training program are listed in Appendix 1.

2.1 *Intermezzo 1:* A Strategy for Failure – or How *Not* to Educate Patients

A physician probably could not be a good doctor or counselor at all if he completely identified with the fate of his patients. This lack of identification is a natural protective mechanism for medical personnel. The result, however, is often that the physician or counselor has no idea of what life is really like for his patients.

The following is a list of examples of how to ensure failure of your education program by conducting it solely from the physician's point of view; in other words, how **not** to conduct a dia betes education program if you do want to take the patient's point of view into account. (The list is incomplete and can be extended indefinitely, of course.)

1. Begin the course by stating that it is still uncertain whether good diabetes control can prevent late complications.
2. At the same time admit the truth: that it is not possible to achieve good control anyway. A mean blood glucose of approx. 120 mg/dl just cannot be compared with a healthy person's (90 mg/dl).
3. Be sure to consistently confuse your patients by using words like "hyperinsulinemia," "peripheral route," "prehepatic" etc., and conclude the chapter with the statement that diabetic patients have too much insulin, anyway, since they inject it. If you want to leave your patients speechless, then just tell them that insulin really should only be administered to the liver's circulatory sphere.
4. During your theoretical discourse on the treatment of diabetes, be sure to emphasize at least in every third or fourth sentence the fact that "it isn't completely proven...," regardless of what you are talking about.
5. If you are conducting the course alone, be sure to set the proper emotional atmosphere. Guard against any show of enthusiasm! Be detached, serious, and above all, skeptical.
6. If you have a teaching team, then be sure there are always new faces (at least seven teachers, one after the other). They should rotate constantly and no one should be specifically responsible for anything. It would be best if the team members did not agree with each other, if they represented different points of view, and (even better!) if they did not even know what their teammates have been talking about.

3 Basic Diabetes Education (Phase I of Rehabilitation)

This chapter briefly outlines the material we feel should be included in the basic diabetes education program. If he is to act responsibly, the patient should have a well-grounded knowledge of his disease and its treatment. In order to increase the acceptability of FIT to the patients and help them "get on with it" as quickly as possible, however, our group tries to make it a policy to dispense with any unnecessary information, especially during this phase of the training program. The emphasis is on knowledge that will be the foundation for putting FIT into practice.

3.1 Insulin Action in Healthy Persons; Insulin Deficiency

Both the function of insulin (glucose transport) as well as the process of insulin secretion that guarantees normal blood sugar (within a range from 75–160 mg/dl) in healthy persons (see Waldhäusl et al. 1979, 1982) should be described, but in the form of a teaching discussion rather than a lecture. The following points are important.

"Basal" insulin secretion in the fasting state (which essentially represents the transport of glucose from hepatic glucose production) is approx. one unit per hour (or 0.35 IU per kg body weight per 24 hours) in healthy persons.

Prandial insulin secretion depends primarily on the amount and also partially on the type of carbohydrates consumed, but to a certain degree on the amount of other nutrients as well. Pran dial secretion in healthy persons is about 1.35 IU insulin per 50 kcal of a glucose equivalent (approx. 12 g carbohydrates, one carbohydrate unit), and about 20% of this amount for the same number of calories in the form of noncarbohydrate nutrients (i.e., 0.45 IU per 100 kcal of noncarbohydrates), since protein or fat consumption will increase hepatic glucose production).

For patients who inject insulin, it is important to consider the events which take place during **physical activity.** In the healthy person, insulin secretion decreases and hepatic glucose production increases. By contrast, in the insulin-treated diabetic patient with good glycemic control, physical activity may lead to an increase in the rate of insulin absorption and in insulin levels, which would disproportionately increase glucose utilization and decrease hepatic glucose production (Vranic and Berger 1979). Only in patients with insulin deficiency does physical activity lead to a further increase in ketosis and hyperglycemia (Berger et al. 1977).

The effects of **alcohol consumption** on insulin secretion should receive special attention. In healthy persons alcohol intake leads to lowered insulin secretion, due to a reduction in hepatic glucose production (Field et al. 1963). When insulin has been injected, the reduction in hepatic glucose production results in a disproportionately high peripheral insulin level, since the peripheral insulin level cannot be abruptly reduced (Chantelau et al. 1985b).

Both physical activity and alcohol intake will thus lead to hypoglycemia in insulin-treated patients unless countermeasures are taken.

The causes and symptoms of insulin deficiency, i.e., of hyperglycemia, glucosuria (dehydration) and acidosis, should be discussed in light of symptoms experienced by the patients themselves. Patients need to be made aware of the long-term results of relative insulin deficiency (i.e., of chronic hyperglycemia), but the diabetes counselor should realize that fear of late complications is not particularly effective in motivating patients to change their behavior (see Sect. 4.4). Some of the particular characteristics of diabetes, such as the fact that patients cannot usually recognize moderate hyperglycemia on the basis of symptoms, should also be discussed in this connection.

The mechanisms which influence glucose homeostasis in healthy persons can be divided into three categories. This allows discussion of ways to substitute insulin according to function and thus of **the principles of functional insulin treatment (FIT):**

1. **Basal insulin secretion** can be replaced by delayed-acting insulins or continuous insulin infusion.

2. **Prandial insulin secretion** can be replaced by preprandial administration of regular (soluble) insulin, or by bolus administration to supplement continuous insulin infusion.
3. The **blood glucose sensor** of the beta cell, which automatically prevents deviation of blood glucose values in the healthy person, can be replaced, although not very satisfactorily at present, by blood glucose self-monitoring with immediate correction of values that deviate from the current target level.

3.2 Diet

One of the most important components of FIT is the patient's ability to administer the correct amount of insulin needed to cover his nutrient intake each time he eats.

3.2.1 Goals of Dietary Counseling

By the end of Phase I the patient should have acquired the ability to correctly estimate the carbohydrate content of the foods he eats. This is absolutely necessary for choosing the correct insulin dose. Although the noncarbohydrate content also has an influence on prandial insulin requirement, this is so small as to be negligible, except when meals are very low in carbohydrates.

The desirable proportion of carbohydrates in the diabetic diet is still the subject of controversy, (Lindsay et al. 1984), although a low fat, high fiber (and therefore high carbohydrate) diet certainly seems to offer the most advantages (Simpson et al. 1981). Throughout the history of diabetes diets, both before and after the discovery of insulin, various combinations have been recommended (Oyen et al. 1985). Today's standpoint has been most concisely formulated by Nuttal (1983): "At the present time, our knowledge regarding the metabolic consequences of various dietary regimens is incomplete and in need of further research. In addition, the composition of various dietary regimens for diabetic persons that will result in the best blood glucose control is uncertain and controversial. Whether dietary changes can significantly delay or prevent the long-term complications of diabetes is also not known. Thus, the insistence that certain foods be avoided by the diabetic person or that a specified diet be adhered to can not be defended scientifically. In view of the above limitations in our knowledge, perhaps the best approach should be to allow diabetic persons to select their own diet and daily plan, as long as the nutrient content is adequate."

This is still valid today. Changes in insulin therapy since 1983 now make it possible to call a second part of Nuttal's statement into question, however: "A diabetic person being treated with insulin...has to comply with a dietary regimen consistent in carbohydrate content and time of meal ingestion. This continues to be of vital importance in the management plan."

Both our own experiences and those of other groups (e. g., Chantelau et al. 1982, 1985a) have shown that functional insulin treatment allows considerable flexibility in regard to quantity and timing of food intake without detracting from the quality of metabolic control. **It is just this possibility of varying the diet, and thus being able to eat – i. e., to be** – like others, that represents the most important factor in the long-term motivation of patients.

A further goal of dietary counseling is for the patient to learn to keep his body weight stable. One of the fears most often expressed by physicians is that patients might abuse the freedom FIT offers by eating more and gaining weight. In our experience it is rather the freedom to eat less – or sometimes not at all – that patients appreciate most. However, we do emphasize the importance of reaching and maintaining normal or ideal body weight.

3.2.2 Estimating the Carbohydrate Content of Food

An exchange system consisting of carbohydrate portions or units uniformly containing approximately 12 g (recently reduced to 10 g) of carbohydrate (regardless of type of carbohydrate) has traditionally been used for planning diabetes diets in Austria and Germany. Since 1 g of carbohydrate contains slightly more than 4 kilocalories, 1 carbohydrate unit (12 g) is approximately equivalent to 50 kcal. Patients are given exchange lists showing the amounts of various foods in grams (with practical descriptions of household-measured quantities), which are equivalent to one carbohydrate unit. About 80% of type I diabetic persons in Austria and Germany have at least some experience with this system.

The guidelines for prandial insulin substitution given in this book are therefore based on these 12 g carbohydrate (CHO) units. As will be shown in Chap. 4, "FIT Training, Phase II of Rehabilitation," each patient develops an individual algorithm for calculating the amount of insulin he needs to inject per carbohydrate unit. Patients who are familiar with an exchange system consisting of 10 g carbohydrate units may simply substitute these in the algorithms, with corresponding mathematical adaptations.

We recommend that all patients learn to calculate carbohydrates in units rather than in grams. Units are easier to conceptualize and more manageable in calculation. For practical purposes, we find that it is most useful to work with the 12 g CHO unit, since it is equivalent to 50 kcal.

In accordance with our policy of dispensing with any unnecessary or irrelevant information, we would not introduce complex exchange lists of food groups (e.g., milk group, bread group, fruit group, etc.), especially if they do not contain equivalent amounts of carbohydrates. Such food exchange groups are helpful in planning an overall balanced diet, but they detract from the important goal during this phase, which is for the patient to learn to calculate the amount of carbohydrates he eats in a way that allows easy estimation of the appropriate insulin dose.

If patients are already adept at using a food group exchange system, they certainly may continue to use it to plan their meals if they wish. Such patients should be able to learn to calculate the total amount of carbohydrate units in a given meal without too much trouble, however.

3.2.3 Prandial Insulin Requirement in Relation to Type and Quantity of Food

The minimum knowledge a patient must have in order to make acceptable decisions as to prandial insulin dose under FIT is simply the answer to the question, "How many units of regular insulin do I need for one carbohydrate unit (12 g CHO)?" Although it is clear that the type of carbohydrate consumed influences prandial insulin requirements, we have not found it helpful to take this into account at this stage of the training program. During phase I, therefore, we touch only globally on absorption rates of carbohydrates in relation to problems that may arise during this phase, and do not recommend classifying foods into groups based on type of carbohydrate or glycemic index (Jenkins et al. 1982).

Later, during phase II, in which patients are trained in the functional use of insulin (see Sect. 5.2, "Prandial insulin substitution. Problems in dosing regular insulin"), they do learn that prandial insulin requirements for rapidly absorbed carbohydrates which cause quick rises in blood glucose are higher than they would be for carbohydrates that affect blood glucose more moderately. They also learn that the least amount of insulin is needed for slowly absorbed foods that produce only a slow rise in blood glucose.

One of the areas which should be discussed in phase I (i.e., before introducing FIT), is eating sweets, since mistakes are likely to lead to complications. Eating sweets is possible under FIT, but – just as for nondiabetic persons – should not be routine. Furthermore, not only does it need a certain degree of experience in FIT, but it is usually almost impossible to estimate the carbohydrate content precisely enough to choose the correct insulin dose. In addition, it is difficult to coordinate the rate of absorption of the insulin injected with that of the carbohydrates consumed. The resulting postprandial hyperglycemia could lead the patient to overcorrect with regular insulin.

As mentioned in Sect. 3.1, the problem of the effects of alcohol should also be discussed as soon as possible. Wine-drinking is common in many cultures and is practically unavoidable at certain social occasions. Some carbohydrate exchange tables *falsely* list a large glass of wine (1/4 liter = approx. 8 oz.) as containing 1 carbohydrate unit (12 g), although dry wines contain practica lly no carbohydrates. Due to the inhibition of hepatic glucose production, insulin requirement is even reduced after the consumption of alcohol without accompanying carbohydrates, and patients need to be made aware of the danger of hypoglycemia. Alcohol consumption in any quantity is certainly not to be recommended, particularly because of the dangers of losing control. But if patients do decide to drink it, they need to know enough to increase their carbohydrate intake accordingly (Chantelau et al. 1985b).

Not only the type of carbohydrate, but also the method of preparation and composition of the meal influences the rate of absorption. This results in certain consequences for prandial insulin dosage which are touched on briefly in phase I and discussed in detail in phase II. After the introduction of FIT, the noncarbohydrate component usually needs to be considered only if the meal is relatively low in carbohydrates. For example, if no prandial insulin is injected, meals consisting of cottage cheese, steak, low-carbohydrate soy bread, etc., would indeed lead to a rise in blood sugar, albeit a slow one, under the conditions of "low" fasting insulin dosage that are recommended under FIT (see Sect. 5.1, "Basal substitution"). The algorithm for these rare situations is obtained by answering the question, "How much regular insulin do I need for 100 kcal of fat/protein in a low-carbohydrate meal?" *Insulin requirements for meals that are low in carbohydrates are only one-sixth (10–20%) of requirements for isocaloric amounts of carbohydrates.* In contrast, the addition of protein, and particularly fat, to a high carbohydrate meal can even reduce prandial insulin requirement by slowing nutrient absorption. Thus, with the usual relatively high carbohydrate diet and a normal amount of protein and fat, the noncarbohydrate component does not need to be considered when calculating insulin dose.

In phase II of the rehabilitation process, patients not only learn how to carry out fine adjustments in insulin amount, but also how to produce changes in the absorption kinetics of prandial insulin to accommodate changes in meal size and composition, physical activity, and even time of day (see Sect. 5.2, "Prandial Substitution. Problems in Dosing Regular Insulin").

3.2.4 Counting Calories and Maintaining Body Weight

Although the ability to estimate the caloric content of food is not absolutely necessary for carrying out FIT, it does provide certain advantages which make the effort worthwhile. We decided to teach our patients to at least roughly estimate calories, not only because they occasionally need a basis to calculate the insulin dose for carbohydrate-free foods, but also because we have found it to be useful in weight reduction and maintenance. The beginning of FIT is often associated with the end of a catabolic state of metabolism. Many patients gain weight because they are no longer losing calories through glucosuria (DCCT-Research Group 1993), so to avoid weight gain they must reduce caloric intake.

The problem of overweight plays a not inconsiderable role in today's society, and well-controlled type I diabetic patients are no exception. For overweight patients, balancing nutrient intake and lowering caloric content is a necessity. Where this is a concern, we feel that in addition to estimating carbohydrates, patients should learn to estimate caloric content of foods. Some therapists prefer to give their overweight patients diet plans or lists of recommended foods vs. foods to avoid. In our experience, however, long-term motivation is greater when patients learn to make their own choices and to compensate for any high-calorie selection. This can be most successfully accomplished within the framework of a behavior modification program in which calorie counting is used as a self-monitoring technique.

Calories are counted on the basis of the following categories: carbohydrates (4 kcal/g), protein (4 kcal/g), fat (9 kcal/g), fiber (theoretically 0 kcal/g), and alcohol (7 kcal/g). About half of the total daily caloric intake (approx. 25–35 kcal/kg body weight) should be in the form of carbohydrates.

For patients who can calculate carbohydrates correctly, but who are incapable of counting calories, we suggest the concept of "sandwich units." It can be assumed that carbohydrates are usually accompanied by an equivalent amount of calories in the form of noncarbohydrates, so that one "sandwich unit" would have about 50 calories from carbohydrates (12 g carbohydrate is equivalent to 50 kcal) and 50 calories from noncarbohydrates. Thus, a "sandwich unit" would contain about 100 calories altogether.

3.2.5 Teaching Tips

Weighing food is essential in learning to estimate carbohydrate and caloric content correctly. It is neither practicable nor necessary, however, to always weigh food in everyday life, as long as the patient has adequate practice in visually estimating amounts. During the training program patients should therefore use a precision diet scale as often as possible (preferably at every meal) so that they can monitor their dietary knowledge and estimating ability. Most people's memories are visual, so learning the carbohydrate unit system can be facilitated by pictorial representation, e.g., pictures of foods in the amounts equivalent to one carbohydrate unit (12 g CHO).

A good way of checking dietary knowledge at the beginning of the program is to lead a group discussion on diet and to ask participants for **examples** of foods equivalent to specified amount of carbohydrates (e.g., one carbohydrate unit) or non-carbohydrates (e.g., 100 kcal of protein or fat).

3.2.6 Problems in Dietary Counseling

The most common mistakes in dietary counseling are: (1) failing to give opportunities for practical experience; (2) making the material too complex (e.g., classifying carbohydrates in too many categories); and (3) demanding an unnecessarily high level of precision, for example, in counting calories. The ability to estimate to within approx. 100 kcal is certainly sufficient.

Teaching methods are also often inadequate. Experience shows that formal lectures on diet are not particularly helpfulbecause they do not allow active participation of the individual,yet they are often used. Carrying out dietary counseling in the form of group discussion provides opportunities both for active participation and for checking the knowledge of group members. For example, each individual group member can be asked for his own estimates of the carbohydrate and/ or energy content of various foods.

Further tips for successful teaching are given in Appendix 1.

3.3 Self-monitoring

Self-monitoring of metabolic parameters is of decisive importance in all forms of insulin therapy, but it is an absolute must for FIT. During phase I of rehabilitation, i.e., before introducing functional insulin treatement, patients should become proficient in determining and evaluating blood glucose as well as glucose and acetone in the urine.

3.3.1 Self-monitoring of Blood Glucose and Targets for Glycemic Control

Phase I of rehabilitation, i.e., basic diabetes education, usually introduces systematic self-adaptation of insulin dosage within the framework of a "split and mixed regular and NPH or lente regimen" (Skyler et al. 1981). In order to reach near-normal levels of hemoglobin A1c (a parameter of long-term glycemic control) with a conventional diabetes diet, at least 4 blood glucose tests are needed per day (Schiffrin et al. 1982a). The number of measurements that are necessary per day for near-normoglycemia under FIT depends on the metabolic stability of the patient, his ability to recognize hypoglycemia, his lifestyle, and many other factors. With variable food intake, provided that the patient has received adequate training in FIT, the number of measurements necessary to normalize HbA_{1c} also seems to be in the vicinity of 4–5 per day. If the patient has mastered proper techniques for drawing blood, this number is well-tolerated.

For didactic reasons, the number of measurements *during the structured group education program* (i.e., phases I and II of rehabilitation, which comprise several days each) should be abou 10–12 per day! It must be emphasized that this number of measurements is only necessary during the training program (see below).

Blood glucose (BG) is monitored at the following times during phases I and II:

- before each meal
- 1–2 hours after each meal
- at bedtime
- at 3 or 4 a.m.
- upon waking (fasting)

After completion of phase II (the structured group training program in FIT), the number of necessary measurements can be reduced to 4–5 per day. For example, for patients with near-normal HbA_{1c}, it is not always necessary to test blood glucose before each meal. Under outpatient conditions, the bedtime value is of the greatest importance. It generally forms the sole basis for decisions which influence the course of blood glucose throughout the period of sleep – which is, after all, approximately one-third of a patient's life.

Fasting blood glucose is also very important, especially since insulin requirement is often elevated early in the morning (Bolli and Gerich 1984; see Sect. 5.1.2, "Fasting Hyperglycemia and Compensation of Circadian Variation in Insulin Requirements"). At least two further blood glucose measurements per day are recommended to keep HbA_{1c} close to the upper limit of the normal range. One-third or more of all measurements should be made randomly 1–2 hours after eating (particularly after breakfast).

Blood glucose monitoring offers the patient relatively accurate information about the actual state of glycemia. In spite of this distinct advantage, it does have two disadvantages when compared to monitoring urine glucose:

1. Drawing blood can be painful, and
2. Blood glucose strips cost more than urine glucose strips.

Since accurate information on actual blood glucose levels is absolutely necessary for FIT, patients need to learn how to cope with these problems. Particularly when a patient is just learning to monitor blood glucose, we have found it helpful to have him use a finger-pricking device in order to make the process as painless as possible. Such devices help in overcoming initial inhibitions about inflicting pain on oneself and also allow blood to be drawn easily from the dominant hand.

The high price of the blood glucose test strips is not a great problem for patients in Austria (although it may be a burden for the health insurance system), since the costs are at present covered, at least for type I diabetic patients, by the obligatory health insurance carriers. Where patients contribute privately to the cost of blood sugar monitoring, it is possible to cut the strips lengthwise so that 2 visually evaluated measurements can be made with one strip.

The patient's techniques of drawing blood should be observed by the trainer and simplified as far as possible. It is important that patients use the fingers of both hands, that they prick only the sides of their fingertips and, if they do not use an automatic finger-pricking device, that they use very fine injection needles rather than lancets, in order to keep the size of the puncture to a minimum. As is the case for insulin injections, prior disinfection of the skin is unnecessary.

In order to increase the practicability of blood glucose monitoring in daily life, the equipment used should be as convenient as possible. For example, it is easier to use test strips that do not need to be rinsed in water. If convenient glucose meters are not available, or if patients

▷

Graphic representation of blood glucose in the form of a curve (Bernstein 1981) has not proven useful. Many of the booklets commonly used for recording "self-variation of insulin dosage" (Berger 1983a) are not particularly suitable for FIT, with its complete flexibility of food intake, because they do not make clear the dynamic relationships with the course of blood glucose over time.

The values for calories are cumulative and include both carbohydrates (1 CHO unit = 50 carbohydrate kcal) and non-carbohydrates. Calorie counting is recommended, but optional, although we do ask it of patients who need to restrict food intake, for example, to lose weight.

The algorithm for insulin dosage for non-carbohydrates should be used only for low-carbohydrate meals.

International Study Group on
Functional Insulin Treatment

PATIENT:
Name: ....
Birth date: .... Tel.: ....
Address: ....
Diabetes since: .... Wt.: ....

Functional insulin treatment (FIT) since .... ○ with injections ○ with pump

INSULIN
- BASAL (fasting requirement): a.m. .... / .... U
- p.m. .... U
- PRANDIAL (meal-related): 1 CHO unit (12g)= .... U
- Correction:

Target for correction of aberrant BG values
Fasting/pre-meal: 100 mg/dl (or .....)
After meals: 1 hour < 160 mg/dl (or < ......)
Target range for MBG: from ...... to ...... mg/dl

1 U regular ins. lowers my BG by approx. .... mg/dl; 1 CHO unit (12g carbohydrates) raises my BG by approx. .... mg/dl

EXAMPLE: Diet (CHO units) ....
Insulin (U) ....

Date:

TIME:		1	2	3	4	5	6	7	8	9	10	11	12	1	2	3	4	5	6	7	8	9	10	11	12	Total
		a.m.												p.m.												
Mon.	Delayed ins.																									
	Regular ins.																									
	BG																									MBG
	CHO																									
	kcal																									
Comments:																										
Tue.	Delayed ins.																									
	Regular ins.																									
	BG																									MBG
	CHO																									
	kcal																									
Comments:																										
Wed.	Delayed ins.																									
	Regular ins.																									
	BG																									MBG
	CHO																									
	kcal																									
Comments:																										
Time:		1	2	3	4	5	6	7	8	9	10	11	12	1	2	3	4	5	6	7	8	9	10	11	12	Total
Thu.	Delayed ins.																									
	Regular ins.																									
	BG																									MBG
	CHO																									
	kcal																									
Comments:																										
Fri.	Delayed ins.																									
	Regular ins.																									
	BG																									MBG
	CHO																									
	kcal																									
Comments:																										
Sat.	Delayed ins.																									
	Regular ins.																									
	BG																									MBG
	CHO																									
	kcal																									
Comments:																										
Sun.	Delayed ins.																									
	Regular ins.																									
	BG																									MBG
	CHO																									
	kcal																									
Time:		1	2	3	4	5	6	7	8	9	10	11	12	1	2	3	4	5	6	7	8	9	10	11	12	

Weekly MBG

Fig. 3.1. Record sheet for documentation of insulin dose, blood glucose and food intake.

do not wish to carry one all the time, they should learn to evaluate test strips visually (Mühlhauser 1984). Visual evaluation should be practiced during group education by making parallel measurements with the laboratory.

The target points for correction of hyperglycemia should lie in the upper range of normal values:

- fasting and preprandial, 100 mg/dl
- postprandial, up to 160 mg/dl

Procedures for making actual decisions on insulin dosage in order to reach the defined target are described in Sect. 4.1.

Special problems can occur at the start of blood glucose self-monitoring; for example, patients may experience phobic reactions either to finger-pricking or to high blood sugar. Especially when patients are new to self-monitoring, a psychological block can occur.
Some become terrified of hurting themselves and simply cannot prick their own fingers. Such patients should never be pressured into self-monitoring before they are ready. With plenty of reassurance, the situation usually improves spontaneously within a few days. Automatic finger-pricking devices do much to overcome this problem. Group support can also be very helpful.

For some patients who have repressed their feelings and fears about diabetes and ignored high blood sugar for years, the beginning of blood glucose self-monitoring can be very unpleasant and they may develop a "high blood sugar trauma." Understandably, negative feelings can arise when these patients are finally confronted with the high blood sugar values they have (unconsciously) feared. Such a reaction is most likely to occur when the patient believes there is little he can do about the situation. Blood glucose self-monitoring under conventional insulin therapy, where the patient has little direct influence on immediate blood sugar values, can be particularly unpleasant for this reason. It is therefore important for patients to be assured from the very beginning, that they will soon be able to control their own blood sugar levels themselves.

3.3.2 Self-monitoring of Urine Glucose

Compared to blood glucose, the test for urine glucose is cheaper and painless. Its major disadvantage lies in its limited ability to predict actual glycemic level. It can only indicate whether the kidney threshold for glucose has been surpassed since the last time urine was passed, and it does not differentiate at all between normal blood glucose levels and hypoglycemia. Sporadic tests of urine glucose are not appropriate as a basis for immediate corrections of blood glucose; they do not provide sufficient information for making decisions as to insulin dose or carbohydrate intake which would ensure adequate blood glucose control. For this reason, they are not sufficient as a basis for FIT.

Testing of urine glucose and acetone can be a valuable teaching tool, however, in order to help patien ts conceptualize the relationship between hyperglycemia, insulin deficit, and glucosuria. Patients learn to test their urine for both glucose and acetone during phase I for this reason.

Tests are made at least three times daily in addition to blood sugar measurements. In phase II the kidney threshold is determined both for purely didactic reasons (see Sect. 4.6, "Determining the Kidney Threshold and Testing Algorithms for Correcting Blood Glucose") and in order to increase the predictive value of the urinary glucose tests.

Under outpatient conditions, self-monitoring of urine glucose is of value for FIT only as an adjunct to blood glucose monitoring and only for certain patients, namely, those who show a discrepancy between mean blood glucose values and HbA_{1c}. Patients who have relatively low mean blood glucose values (e.g., below 140 mg/dl), but high glycosylated hemoglobin (more than 1% above the normal limit), for example, may be missing intermittent, postprandially occurring hyperglycemia because blood glucose is being monitored only before meals. We have found it helpful with such patients to have them test **each** urine portion over 1–2 days per week, so that they can see the degree of glucosuria/ketonuria themselves.

Table 3.1. Phase III of rehabilitation: measures for self-monitoring in outpatients after training in FIT

1.	**Blood glucose** (BG)	**Minimum**	**Optimum**
	Number of BG measurements per day?	4	6
	Does patient carry strips?	yes	yes
	At what times are measurements made?	**Priority:**	
	- bedtime	1	
	- fasting	2	
	- daytime - preprandial	3	
	- at least 30% of all measurements 1-2 h postprandially (e.g., after breakfast)	4	
2.	**Ketonuria**	**Minimum**	**Optimum**
	Measurements made?	occasionally: • if BG > 300 mg/dl, or during hypocaloric nutrition	if BG > 240 mg/dl
3.	**Glucosuria**		
3.1	*Optional* • if HbA_{1c} normal • if kidney threshold atypical - higher than 250 or - lower than 140 mg/dl		
3.2	*Obligatory* (exceptional cases) • if HbA_{1c} > 1% above norm and/or • if < 4 BG measurements/day • if BG measurements are preprandial only	**Minimum** once/day	**Optimum** once/day in addition on 1-2 days/wk **all urine portions**

Measures for self-monitoring during FIT-training program (Phase II):

1. **Blood glucose:** As often as possible (at least 8× daily)
2. **Ketonuria:** As often as possible (at least 3× daily)
3. **Glucosuria:** As often as possible (at least 3× daily)
4. **HbA_{1c} (Diabetes Center):** Patient information? (Predictive value, meaning, norms, target value, course, evaluation of compatibility with clinical data.)

3.3.3 Determination of Acetone in Urine

Patients need to know that the presence of acetone in the urine of a type I (insulin-dependent) diabetic person means one of two things: (1) there is an insulin deficit, or (2) a catabolic metabolic situation has resulted from hypocaloric nutrition.

In the overwhelming majority of cases, the cause is insulin deficiency. Ketonuria is always a pathological sign if glucosuria is also present. Testing for acetone in the urine becomes particularly important with continuous insulin infusion, since in case of pump failure the lack of subcutaneous insulin deposits can lead to a relatively rapid development of ketosis.

Independently of form of therapy, urine should be tested for acetone in all situations that might lead to an increase in insulin requirement (hyperglycemia), such as acute illness, surgery, accidents, etc. Patients should therefore be asked to test for acetone in any case if blood glucose is over 300 mg/dl. Patients with insulin pumps should test at values over 240 mg/dl. Checking for acetone in urine can also be valuable for patients with an "insulin phobia," who for psychological reasons tend to keep insulin doses extremely low.

3.3.4 Targets for Glycemic Control

Mean blood glucose (MBG) of the day is best suited for the everyday evaluation of glycemic control by the patient himself. MBG target range between 110 and 160 (170) mg/dl corresponds to the target for HbA_{1c} between the upper limit of normal and about 1,5% above that. However, glycemic targets have to be chosen individually (DDCT Research Group 1993, see Sect. 8.2.4.)

3.4 Strategies for Insulin Treatment

In order to make a decision for a certain form of therapy, the patient needs to be sufficiently informed about the various strategies of insulin treatment currently available. Although the various treatment forms often overlap, we identify several main groups on the basis of certain typical characteristics:

(1) conventional insulin therapy,
(2) intensified insulin therapy, and
(3) functional insulin treatment.

Different strategies (e.g., "split and mixed regular and NPH or lente," "bedtime NPH and three doses of regular," "one or two doses of ultralente and three doses of regular," "continuous subcutaneous infusion") have been included in group 2, "intensified insulin therapy," (Skyler et al. 1981, Schade, Santiago, Skyler, Rizza 1989). Unfortunately, nomenclature varies among countries and even among diabetes centers, making communication between therapists sometimes difficult. In order to clarify the distinctive aspects of FIT, the characteristics of the three groups are summarized in Table 3.2.

In my opinion, the decisive criterion for categorizing the various therapeutic regimes is not the relative degree of effort involved, i.e., not the "intensity" of the treatment. It would be false and misleading to confuse the present form of FIT with its historical precursors (i.e., "ultralente-based insulin regimens," or continuous insulin infusion), which would require constantly regimented diet and lifestyle without allowances for immediate correction of hyperglycemia. Due to the freedom of diet and the capability for immediately influencing blood sugar offered by FIT, taken as a whole, it actually entails less exertion than many other forms of insulin therapy. Thus, the ultimate criterion for classification is *whether and in what way the insulin dosage is contingent on the results of self-monitoring of blood glucose.*

In regard to **insulins**, conventional therapy typically uses intermediate and/or mixed types. Basal and prandial insulin are replaced globally rather than separately. Intensified insulin therapy goes a step further. It uses regular and delayed-acting insulins separately. Occasionally, it does differentiate basal and prandial insulin function to a certain degree, but remains relatively rigid.

Type I Diabetes — Treatment Characteristics / Treatment Strategy	Conventional	Intensified	Functional	
INSULIN				
Kinetics:				
– regular/rapid acting analogs		+	+	
– intermediate	+	(+)	(+)	
– long-acting (ultralente)			+	
Mode of delivery:				
– injections	(+)	(+)	(+)	
– infusion		(+)	(+)	
Function: (basal/prandial/correction)				
– not separate	+	(+)		
– separate		(+)	+	
FLEXIBILITY OF DIET				
– fixed	+			
– flexible		+		
– free (but balanced)			+	
SELF-MONITORING				
Type:				
– blood glucose		(+)	+	
– urine glucose	(+)	(+)		
Frequency:				
– ∅	+			
– often		+	+	
Feedback loop: (Insulin → Self-monitoring → Insulin)				
– ∅	+			
– delayed		+	+	⟵ secondary } adaptation of insulin dose (see "Rules for Algorithm Modification")
– immediate			+	⟵ primary } adaptation of insulin dose (see "Rules for Algorithm Modification")

Table 3.2. Summary of characteristics of various types of insulin strategies. The decisive factor in differentiating between strategies is whether and in what way insulin dosage is based on the results of self-monitoring.

FIT goes even further, providing not only for administration according to basal and prandial function, but also for specific insulin administration to correct any blood glucose excursion. **FIT thus requires functionally differentiated administration of insulin for basal, prandial or corrective purposes.** The use of regular insulin, either for prandial substitution or correction of hyperglyce mia (independently of each other), is therefore absolutely necessary for FIT.

The **method of insulin delivery** is not very useful for differentiating between therapy types. Conventional therapy is most often carried out with injections, but it is also possible (and often done, unfortunately) to simply prescribe an insulin infusion pump with a fixed rate and a fixed diet, giving the patient no opportunity to influence his actual blood glucose level. Although controlled continuous insulin infusion is well-suited to either intensified therapy or FIT, multiple daily injections can be used equally well for both.

In conventional and intensified therapy, **diet** is a consequence of the insulin administered, i.e., the patient must adapt his food intake to accommodate insulin action. In FIT, the insulin a dministered is rather a consequence of diet; i.e., the patient adapts his insulin administration to accommodate his personal lifestyle.

Both intensified insulin therapy and functional insulin substitution require **self-monitoring** (usually of blood glucose). The type of treatment strategy is not determined by the type or fr equency of self-monitoring, however. The decisive factor is whether the self-monitoring has immediate consequences. In conventional insulin therapy, there is practically no feedback loop between self-monitoring results and insulin dosage. With intensified insulin therapy, the reaction is delayed, since changes in insulin dose are usually made only after self-monitored values have shown certain trends or patterns over several days. With functional substitution, however, the patient reacts with immediate corrective measures after every value that deviates from the desired level. In this way he can achieve near-normoglycemia. Thus, FIT is based on glycemia-dependent self-dosage of insulin.

Which regime should patients be advised to choose? If we consider the fact that under classical, conventional insulin therapy, self-monitoring is either not carried out at all, or if it is, then usually without immediate consequences, then it is clear that this type of treatment cannot be recommended for the average insulin-dependent diabetic patient. The real choice is therefore between intensified insulin therapy and functional insulin substitution. Here the patient must make his own decision.

Intensified insulin therapy, in which **at least 2–3 insulin injections are carried out per day, is the absolute minimum in the current long-term treatment of type I diabetes. The patient must also at least be able to make independent decisions as to the amounts of regular and long-acting insulins he injects in the morning and evening.** So defined, insulin dose adaptation is an absolute prerequisite for adequate treatment of type I diabetes today. Intensified therapy also requires that **self-monitoring be carried out at least four times per day** in order to provide information on the glycemic levels obtained during the action of the various insulin components. Since basal and prandial insulin are replaced together in this type of regime (especially if there are only two daily injections), a fixed meal plan suited to the level of insulinemia produced by the insulin mixture must be maintained.

The advantages and disadvantages of intensified insulin therapy versus FIT are discussed extensively in phase I. FIT has two major advantages: (1) it allows variable food intake (regarding not only meal size and composition, but also frequency); (2) near-normoglycemia can be achieved more easily with immediate measures for correcting blood glucose levels.

In our experience these two advantages lead to a corresponding desire in patients to at least try FIT. The biggest drawback as compared to conventional or intensified therapy seems to lie not in the frequency of self-monitoring or of injections, but in the fact that FIT requires the patient to take responsibility for his own glycemic control. Being able to influence (and control) blood glucose also means being obliged to do so. Sufficient information and capability carry with them a degree of responsibility that can sometimes be unpleasant. In contrast, conventional insulin therapy – even an intensified regime – offers the patient the seeming advantages of passivity and passing on responsibility to the medical team. ("I inject the prescribed amount of insulin and stick to the diet, the rest is up to the doctor.") Conventional therapy also makes it easy to repress one's feelings about the disease; since one can't do anything about hyperglycemia, it is better to forget about it.

In our experience, the overwhelming majority (more than 95%) of patients who go through this extensive information phase do decide to take on responsibility for their own therapy and choose FIT, in spite of the drawbacks of frequent insulin injections. In our experience, the few patients who are well-informed, but nonetheless decide for conventional therapy, do so because they do not (yet) feel able to take on so much responsibility for their own treatment. Unwillingness to carry out so many insulin injections is seldom the cause.

3.5 Insulin

3.5.1 Pharmacokinetics

In order to adjust insulin dosage, patients need to understand the dynamics of insulin action. With subcutaneous administration, peak and duration of insulin activity are dose-dependent (the larger the dose, the longer the duration and the later the peak of activity). Both intra- and inter- individual variations in activity characteristics need to be considered.

For intensified insulin treatment (e.g., "split and mixed regimens"), we would recommend shorter-acting delayed insulins and would therefore prefer NPH/isophane to lente insulins for the delayed-acting component.

Under FIT, regular insulin is always used for prandial replacement and correction of out-of-range values. S. Rapid acting analogs will probably be even more suitable for these purposes (see also Appendix 4 and Sect. 5.2): In comparison to regular insulin, insulin Lispro shows an immediate onset of action, peak aktivity within 1 h (regular 2–4 h) and correspondingly shorter duration of action (less than 3 h vs 6–8 h in case of s.c. regular insulin. Basal requirements can be fulfilled either with a delayed-acting insulin or with continuous insulin infusion. Since experience shows that over 90% of patients have a higher basal requirement in the morning, a small amount of regular insulin (approx. 10% of total daily requirement) should be included as a component of the morning dose of basal insulin to compensate for this. The delayed-acting insulins chosen for basal insulinization under FIT should have the longest possible duration of activity and the smoothest possible activity curve **(see Appendix 4)**. Insulins of the following types are suitable if they are administered twice daily: ultralente (duration of relevant activity 18–30 h, depending on dose); lente (14–24 h); and NPH/isophane (10–18 h). On the basis of the results of an intraindividual crossover study in our patients, we currently recommend either an ultralente insulin twice daily or a combination of an ultralente insulin (in the morning) with an NPH/isophane (or a lente insulin) at bedtime. A combination is particularly suitable for patients with a tendency towards early-morning hyperglycemia ("dawn phenomenon"), since these insulins show a more pronounced peak (approx. 5–7 and 6–10 hours post-injection, respectively, depending on dose). Provided that they are injected at bedtime they are capable of eliminating the early-morning insulin deficit. In contrast, due to their protracted action and flat activity curves, it is practically impossible to influence circumscribed time periods with ultralente insulins (see Sect. 5.1.2).

Patients who are well-trained in compensating for irregularities in the basal rate may also use NPH or lente insulins twice daily. An NPH insulin twice daily is the most suitable for blind patients, since NPH insulins are currently the only delayed-acting insulins available for use with insulin pens, which enable the blind patient to administer insulin without help from others.

When injected twice daily, ultralente insulins have the advantage that the time point of the basal injection can be varied by up to 3 or 4 hours. For example, an ultralente insulin can be injected one day at 7 p.m. and the next at 10 p.m. This flexibility results from the overlapping duration of activity and is much appreciated by patients.

We basically recommend that insulins not be mixed in the syringe. However, if keeping the number of daily injections to a minimum is a concern, it has been suggested that an NPH insulin be used to cover basal requirement. In contrast to lente or ultralente (zinc depot) insulins, which may cause changes in the action of regular insulin (due to reduced bio-availability caused by excess zinc) when mixed, NPH insulins can be satisfactorily mixed with regular (soluble) insulin in the same syringe. However, the relatively distinct peak and the shorter duration of activity of NPH – and to a lesser degree of lente – insulins, especially at lower dosage levels, make it hard to produce the uniformity desirable for basal insulinization, at least during the daytime. Most of our patients prefer to use an ultralente insulin to cover basal requirements, at least for the morning dose, in order to avoid the noontime tendency towards hypoglycemia and/or the evening "insulin gap" which may occur with NPH or lente insulins.

Since the switch to FIT usually involves a change in insulin type, anyway, if the patient is not already on human insulin, we prescribe it at this time. This circumvents the possibility that future switches might be made by other treatment centers. Except for the slightly reduced antigenicity, human insulin does not bring any particular advantages, although when the analog animal insulins are used, insulin requirement is slightly (5–10%) higher. The duration of activity of animal insulins (especially of ultralente) is somewhat longer than that of the corresponding human insulins.

3.5.2 Insulin Delivery

Under FIT there are two main methods of insulin delivery: (1) continuous insulin infusion with a programmable insulin pump (under long-term outpatient conditions, only the s.c. route of delivery, the simplest, and the one with the fewest complications, has proven useful); and (2) multiple daily injections of regular insulin (prandial and/or for blood sugar correction) in combination with delayed-acting insulin (twice daily).

The advantage of continuous subcutaneous insulin infusion (CSII) is primarily the excellent basal insulinization, which is especially beneficial for patients with early-morning hyperglycemia. The major disadvantage as compared to multiple daily injections is the necessity of continually wearing the pump, which can lead to a kind of "prosthesis complex." This psychological problem explains the relatively poor acceptance of pump therapy (Teutsch et al. 1984). At most, only 10% of non-pregnant patients can usually be convinced of the advantages of an infusion device. The relatively high price and potential defects also provide grounds for deliberation. Technical failures can potentially stop insulin delivery, causing acute insulin deficiency. Acute metabolic derangement can be avoided, however, even with completely discontinued insulin delivery, if blood sugar is self-monitored with the recommended frequency (at least 3–5 times daily). Many patients complain of problems at the infusion site, although these can be avoided by frequent catheter and cannula changes.

Pumps have proven useful for certain types of patients (especially for the blind), and technical improvements may eliminate many of the problems. When choosing an insulin pump, the following factors need to be considered:

1. Operational simplicity. The simpler the device, the fewer the possible errors.
2. Pattern of prandial insulin delivery. In order to insure adequate postprandial insulinemia, prandial insulin should be given in bolus form within seconds (Sonnenberg 1983), not with a rectangular profile (over minutes or hours).
3. Size of infusion device. This often determines whether a patient will accept CSII. The smallest pumps are naturally preferred.

As compared to CSII, multiple daily injections are more inconspicuous, and therefore socially more acceptable and more widely applicable, especially if a cartridge-filled insulin pen is used rather than a conventional syringe. In our experience, this method is chosen by about 90% of patients, even in an unselected patient group. As compared to CSII, this simple method of insulin delivery not only has the advantage of being less prone to technical difficulties, but also offers the possibility of influencing the speed of insulin absorption according to need, for example, by producing local hyperemia or changing the injection mode, etc. (see Sect. 5.2, "Prandial Insulin Substitution").

One of the disadvantages of multiple daily injections is the pain experienced with poor injection technique, but this can be avoided if proper techniques are learned. Another problem is the possibility of hematoma at the injection site, but most patients are willing to accept this on less exposed parts of the body (e.g., the inner thigh or calves, if there are no varicosities).

3.5.3 Special Aspects of the Practicability of Insulin Delivery

The disadvantages of both multiple injections and the pump can be reduced to a relative minimum if the patient is instructed in appropriate techniques.

• CSII

The practicability and acceptability of CSII depends on whether the pump can be easily concealed. This usually plays a decisive role for the patient. It should therefore be pointed out that a pump could easily and acceptably be worn in the pocket, on a belt under clothing, or inside a brassiere, for example.

- **Multiple Injections**

In our experience, at least half of all patients use an injection technique that is much too complicated. Injections take too long and too much importance is placed on them ("insulin worship"). The patient's injection technique therefore needs to be observed by the trainer and simplified, if necessary. It is especially important to point out any unnecessary components; for example, disinfecting the skin, changing needles at every injection, etc. Since today's insulins contain disinfectants such as phenol or cresol, etc., anyway, as long as the skin is clean, it is not necessary to apply a disinfectant before the injection (Berger et al. 1983a, 1986; our own observations). If a syringe with a fixed needle is used (e.g., Becton-Dickinson MicroFine), multiple use is an absolute necessity from a practical (and financial) standpoint. There is no harm in using it until the needle is dull.

For injections of regular insulin, even patients with average insulin requirements (total daily dose between 30 and 70 IU) find it helpful to use insulin syringes designed especially for low doses (such as used to be common for children). This allows exact dosing in half units. A patient with the above-mentioned insulin requirements would almost never inject more than 8–12 IU of insulin at one time under FIT, although he may well wish to inject half a unit.

An insulin vial or cartridge currently in use can also be stored at room temperature for weeks or even months with no problems (Brange et al. 1987). Refrigeration is only necessary for more lengthy storage.

Some patients develop lipohypertrophy at the injection site. Intramuscular insulin administration seems to protect against lipohypertrophy of the subcutis (our own observation). In order to avoid the nuisance of having to remove clothing several times a day to expose the injection site, regular insulin can certainly be injected into easily accessible body parts, such as the lower arm or the calf.

The antipathy of most patients to frequent injections actually results from historically conditioned misconceptions: for example, that it hurts, it has to be done at a certain time, one has to get undressed, one always needs a new syringe or a new needle, alcohol, swabs, a refrigerator, etc. These associations need to be replaced with appropriate information in order to gain long-term patient acceptance of multiple daily injections.

4 FIT Training (Phase II of Rehabilitation)

The major goal of phase II is to set up and test individualized algorithms (rules) for insulin substitution. The patient learns to use his algorithms to keep his blood glucose level close to his chosen target by correcting off-target blood glucose values (primary adjustment of insulin dosage). He also learns to modify his algorithms as necessary (secondary adjustment). He explores the possibilities of improving his quality of life and tests the limits of functional insulin treatment.

4.1 Initial Algorithms, "K" and the Blood Glucose Target Value

Generating the Initial Algorithms for Functional Insulin Use
The initial algorithms represent rules for dosing insulin according to the three basic functions discussed in Sect. 3.1, "Insulin action in healthy persons; insulin deficiency": (1) replacing basal insulin, (2) compensating for nutrient intake, (3) correcting deviations of blood glucose. They consist of provisional answers to the questions the patient must answer in order to carry out functional insulin treatment (Table 4.1, "How to close the open loop?"). Guidelines for generating the initial algorithms are presented in Table 4.2. In practice, the quality of the initial algorithms for an individual patient usually depends on the experience and intuition of the therapist. The mathematical formulations given here represent an attempt to satisfy a pragmatic desire for a transferable method. An experienced therapist may come up with algorithms that are even better suited to an individual patient. An alternative method of determining algorithms which takes the patient's current level of metabolic control into account is presented in **Appendix 3** in the form of a **nomogram** based on empirical data.

Table 4.1. "How to close the open loop?" Questions the patient asks himself in order to link insulin dosage to blood glucose level.

1. **How high is my basal (fasting) insulin requirement?**
2. **How can I substitute my fasting insulin?**
   In other words,
   - How much of which insulin (and when) should I inject, even if I don't eat?
3. **How high is my prandial insulin requirement for a specified meal?**
   In other words,
   How many units of regular insulin do I need
   - for 12 g of carbohydrates (1 CHO unit = 50 kcal)?
   - for 100 kcal of protein and/or fat (in case of a lowcarbohydrate meal)?
4. **How can I substitute my prandial insulin?**
   In other words,
   - How much of which insulin?
   - How should it be administered?
   - How long should I wait before eating?
5. **How can I influence my blood sugar at a given time?**
   In other words,
   - What is the effect of 1 unit of regular insulin?
   - What is the effect of 1 unit of carbohydrates (12 g CHO, i.e. 50 kcal from carbohydrates)?
6. **What is my blood sugar target level?**

Before changing insulin treatment strategy it is good to know:
- How does my insulin act?
- What changes its kinetics?
- Why is it not advisable to eat if my blood sugar is already high?
- What is my target level for mean blood glucose (MBG)?

The mathematical model (Czerwenka-Howorka et al. 1984) for the initial algorithms for basal insulin substitution and for compensation of carbohydrate intake were derived from data on the insulin production rate of healthy persons (Waldhäusl et al. 1979). The algorithms for correction of blood glucose values that deviate from the target level are based on experience (Skyler et al. 1981; Bernstein 1981) and empirical data, as are the equations for the algorithms for prandial insulin to compensate for protein and fat (van Halle et al. 1981; Bernstein 1981) taken at low-carbohydrate meals.

Table 4.2. Initial algorithms of FIT: An attempt at pragmatic description of therapeutic experience.

Basal insulin:* 0.35 IU × K × body wt in kg / 24 h

Prandial insulin:

for 12 g (50 kcal) carbohydrates:	1.35 IU × K
for 100 kcal protein/fat mixture: (low carbohydrate meals only)	0.45 IU × K

Correction of blood glucose values outside target range:
Change in blood glucose (delta BG) in mg/dl per:

$$1\text{ IU regular insulin} = -35 \times \frac{1}{K} \times \frac{60}{\text{kg body wt}}$$

$$1\text{ carbohydrate unit (12 g CHO)} = +50 \times \frac{60}{\text{kg body wt}}$$

Blood glucose target:

Fasting and preprandial	= 100 mg/dl
1 h postprandial	< 160 mg/dl
2 h postprandial	< 140 mg/dl

Intervals between consecutive corrections of blood glucose must not be less than 3 hours.
Target range for MBG: 100 (120)–160 (180) mg/dl

K (an empirically determined, clinical correction factor which describes individual insulin sensitivity):

$$K = \frac{\text{current insulin requirement (IU/24 h)}}{\text{theoretical insulin requirement** (IU/24 h)}}$$

A nomogram for developing the initial algorithms of FIT based on current insulin dose per 24 hours and level of glycemic control is given in Appendix 3.

* If long-acting insulin is used instead of an insulin infusion pump, about 10% more insulin is needed.
** From Waldhäusl et al. 1979.

The K Quotient

Individual differences in insulin sensitivity in diabetic patients are taken into account by means of a factor called K. This is a quotient that is calculated by dividing the mean current total daily insulin dose (assuming a reasonable level of metabolic control) by the theoretical daily insulin requirement, which is derived from studies on endogenous insulin requirements in healthy persons (Waldhäusl et al. 1979). Thus, K is based on average daily insulin requirement and corresponds to a clinical correction factor which describes individual insulin sensitivity Table 4.2). It can be assumed that a C-peptide positive patient with some remaining residual function would have a K value smaller than 1. A patient with no residual function and no insulin resistance would have a K value equal to 1, and a patient with insulin resistance would have a K value greater than 1.

The Blood Glucose Target and Use of Insulin for Correction
The target value for blood glucose should lie close to the upper range of normal values. In making actual decisions on insulin dosage, the target must be defined as **a point** within this range (with differing preprandial and postprandial target points), since it is used as a **reference value to calculate** whether there is currently an insulin deficit and **how much insulin is neede for correction.** Thus, for most patients, the target values would be:

- 100 mg/dl for fasting and preprandial blood glucose
- up to 160 (180) mg/dl for postprandial blood glucose.

Correction of above-target values should be undertaken if there is an insulin deficit of 1–2 U; i.e., if the patient calculates on the basis of his algorithm for blood glucose correction that he would have to inject more than 1–2 U of insulin to reach his target level. The minimum time interval between consecutive corrections of hyperglycemia must not be less than about three hours. (The time interval between correction and last prandial injection can be shorter, however.) Using insulin for **correction should be independent of prandial insulin replacement,** although, if appropr iate, it can be also be carried out with the same injection. In any case, it is not necessary to make corrections only before meals.

In order to avoid hypoglycemia, we consider any blood glucose values under 90 mg/dl in nonpregnant diabetic patients to be below target and thus in need of correction. In 20–40% of cases, the above-mentioned target values are modified because of special circumstances or patient characteristics (e.g., hypoglycemia unawareness, pregnancy, etc.; see Chap. 8, "Rules for Modifying Algorithms").

Practical Aspects of Setting Up the Initial Algorithms
The basal insulin requirement can be substituted either with an insulin infusion device or with twice-daily injections of delayed-acting

insulin. With either method, a slight amount of regular (soluble) insulin is usually necessary in the morning (an average of 4 IU of regular insulin, or about 10% of total daily requirement) in order to compensate for increased requirements in the morning. This is considered to be part of the basal requirement (see Sect. 5.1, "Basal insulin").

Only regular insulin can be used for fulfilling the prandial insulin requirement and correcting blood glucose excursions. Various techniques may be used in order to achieve an adequate level of postprandial insulinemia without increasing the dose. For example, the interval between injecting and eating could be lengthened, although this is often not feasible. Alternatively, modifications could be made in insulin absorption kinetics; e.g., by means of intramuscular injections, local hyperemia, or rapid acting analogs (see Sect. 5.2, "Prandial substitution. Problems in dosing regular insulin"). Such measures can also be used when correcting blood glucose excursions.

The initial algorithms are defined by the physician or the trainer. They are then applied, tested and – if necessary – modified by the patient under the physician's or trainer's guidance. Here the question arises as to how important it is for the initial algorithms to be "correct," or whether it matters if they need modification. On the one hand, it is important that they be as accurate as possible in order to give the patient confidence in his trainer and enable him to enjoy the feeling of being in control of his blood sugar levels as soon as possible. On the other hand, it really does not matter if the initial algorithms are not correct, since the experience of evaluating them and deciding which are inappropriate and how they should be modified is equally valuable.

4.2 *Intermezzo 2:* A Strategy for Failure, or How to Demotivate Even the Most Convinced Enthusiast

Let us return to our ever-expanding collection of evidence that FIT cannot possibly be accepted or practiced by patients:

1. The first thing to do to guarantee failure is to point out everything that the "absolutely have to do," for example:
   - Eat regular meals (6–7 small meals per day, with no exceptions)
   - Inject insulin every time they eat
   - Maintain a fixed interval between injecting and eating (just to make sure, don't tell them why)
   - Test their blood sugar every single time they eat.
2. Be sure to demand the highest level of accuracy. Special emphasis should be put on counting calories exactly. For example, 123 g of sausage has 327 kcal. Make sure patients know they will have to do this for the rest of their lives. Be sure to complicate the introduction of carbohydrates. Especially patients who have no previous knowledge need to learn to classify carbohydrates in at least five or more categories. This method ensures that patients do not dare to eat anything at all, which of course makes the control of diabetes much easier.
3. Emphasize that the algorithms also need to be as accurate as possible, at least to the second decimal place. For example, 1.46 IU of insulin for every 12.52 g of carbohydrates consumed, etc. Don't forget to explain the concept of the K value in exhaustive detail, especially to patients with the lowest level of education and the least imagination. If there is a general lack of understanding, distribute brochures containing the scientific formulas that describe the theoretical background of insulin sensitivity.
4. Emphasize to the patient the importance of always using a glucose meter when monitoring blood glucose and of carrying it with him wherever he goes. He should never trust his own visual judgment, since retinopathy may cause him to see blue instead of green, and vice versa.
5. Should the patient be against multiple injections at first, you must tell him that he absolutely needs an infusion pump instead. Especially visually handicapped patients should choose a nice complex pump with at least 4 different basal rates and a sufficiently complicated multirectangular profile for prandial insulin with exponential increments that can be called up digitally. Models with suitable acoustic signals and short catheters have been found useful in preventing patients from having satisfactory sexual lives. Do not in any circumstances discuss the possibility of removing the pump for short periods of time, since this entails the risk that the patient may actually do so.

6. We have already noted the importance of maintaining the proper emotional attitude towards both patients and the material you are presenting. (Beware of showing enthusiasm!) In addition to the tried and true method of skeptical indifference ("...Firstly, we don't know whether this does any good, and secondly, no one manages to do it, anyway..."), two further methods of training seem to meet with similar success. One is the "overdemanding-contradictory method" ("...During pregnancy you must keep your mean blood sugar at about 50 mg/dl, but you must not have any hypoglycemic episodes!..."). The other is the "dramatic-compulsive method," in which the trainer begins to sob when a patient reports high blood glucose values, say around 300 mg/dl, and then drastically alters all the patient's algorithms immediately (without asking for any explanations or suggestions from the patient), documenting the change on the patient's protocol in red – just to be sure....
7. Or you can do it the comfortable way.... Just give the patient an insulin pen and say with a convincing smile, "From now on you can eat anything you want...," then close the discussion. If the patient should ask how to dose the insulin, just reply with the brief statement, "You'll see."

4.3 Introducing FIT in Practice

For psychodynamic reasons, the introduction of functional insulin treatment should be abrupt. Just as one cannot be "a little bit pregnant," one cannot do "a little bit of FIT." The therapist cannot delegate the responsibility for blood glucose levels to the patient without simultaneously delegating responsibility for diet and self-variation of insulin dose as well. This means, however, that from the moment the patient takes over the responsibility for his glycemic control, he must be sufficiently trained and emotionally prepared to handle it. FIT cannot be achieved just by changing insulins or simply prescribing multiple injections or a pump. **The decisive factor is the ability and will of the patient to control his blood glucose.**

How can we decide when the time is right for handing over the responsibility for actual glycemia to the patient? It is helpful to judge on the basis of the patient's:

(1) information status,
(2) skills, and
(3) motivation for active and self-responsible action.

The patient's **information status** is adequate when he can answer the following questions (see Table 4.1, "How to close the open loop?"): How can I substitute my fasting insulin? How can I substitute my prandial insulin? How can I correct blood sugar levels that are too high or too low? The minimum knowledge the patient must have includes the basic facts about insulin action, diet and self-monitoring that were presented in phase I.

The patient cannot begin FIT without certain **practical skills.** He must be able to calculate the amount of the actual insulin deficit. Besides knowing his own algorithms, the patient must also have mastered basic arithmetic. Be sure to check this in time. You can see how things stand by assigning a few simple exercises; for example, "If you need two units of insulin to take care of one carbohydrate unit, how much insulin do you need for three carbohydrate units?" Or, "Assume you have measured your blood sugar and it is 200 mg/dl, although your target (before eating) is 100 mg/dl. If you need one unit of regular insulin to lower your blood sugar by 40 mg/dl, how many units of insulin do you still need to correct your blood sugar?" In our experience one needs at least an hour for working out such exercises in the group on the day before beginning functional insulin substitution.

The patient must also have mastered the techniques of self-monitoring before he can start with the new strategy. If he has an emotional block which prevents him from pricking his finger for the blood glucose test, he is not ready to begin FIT. If he has a glucose meter, you must also be sure he knows how to use it properly. The same goes for an insulin infusion device.

The third, probably most important criterion for beginning FIT is sufficient **motivation** on the part of the patient. This is an absolute prerequisite. If the patient is not convinced that he wants to actively make decisions and take control of his blood sugar on his own, then FIT will not work. You can recognize a truly motivated patient by his curiosity, impatience to begin, and by the questions he asks. It does not seem advisable to try to persuade patients who seem passive, indifferent or depressed to carry out FIT. They may be interested later. Some may need to work through specific individual problems first.

Patients who have completed phase I of the rehabilitation processare now theoretically capable of dosing insulin on the basis of their individual algorithms. In practice, however, it is advisable to discuss with them what they plan to eat and help them calculate the necessary prandial doses for the first day. For the time being, it is also best to advise them to use the correction algorithm only for correcting pre-prandial blood glucose values. In the beginning, many tend to over-correct high values; for example, they may give themselves a second correcting dose postprandially without waiting long enough for the first correction to take effect.

The trainer should not place too much importance on occasional blood glucose values that are too high or too low. At the beginning of FIT **the goal is not so much to obtain good blood sugar va lues as such, as it is to teach the patient to analyze the causes of any values that are too high or too low and to be able to remove them himself** (see Chap. 6, "Hypoglycemia," and Chap. 7, "Hyperglycemia").

Responsibility for controlling actual blood glucose gives rise to an important guiding principle of FIT (see also Bernstein 1981): "If your blood sugar is elevated, lower it with regular insulin **before** eating." Hyperglycemia means acute insulin deficiency. Although patients may decide to eat for other (emotional) reasons, there is no rational reason for further nutrient intake while hyperglycemia. In spite of extensive diabetes education programs, it is amazing how rarely this simple fact is pointed out to patients. From now on the patient can correct blood sugar with regular insulin (admittedly it will take him a while to come down, for example, from 250 mg/dl to normal values, even with regular insulin). The only logical way is first to normalize blood sugar, i.e., to remove the acute insulin deficiency in order to compensate for the oversupply of nutrients *before* replenishing the nutrients. The first day under the new insulin strategy is an excellent opportunity for the discussion of this principle: "If your blood sugar is high, don't eat. Lower it first!"

Patients who choose multiple daily injections rather than CSII may have some trouble at first with the number of necessary injections. If the traditional diabetes diet with 6–7 meals per day is maintained, this would mean at least 8–9 injections per day. Especially at the beginning, one solution is to take care of two meals (for example, one main meal and a snack) with one injection. However, this means that the patient must eat the planned snack in order to avoid hypoglycemia. Most patients prefer to reduce the number of meals they take to about 4 (3–5) per day.

When treatment with ultralente insulins was first introduced, a so-called loading dose, i.e., the initial administration of substantially higher doses of long-acting insulin than would be necessary as a maintenance dose, was suggested in order to obtain a sufficient level of insulinemia as soon as possible (Phillips et al. 1979; Turner et al. 1982). We have not found this helpful when beginning FIT. The reason is that the idea of the loading dose was conceived within the framework of a fixed insulin strategy, where the patient did not make any immediate corrections of hyperglycemic values. Under FIT, the patient is capable of immediately removing any acute insulin deficit (i.e., correcting hyperglycemia) with an appropriate dose of regular insulin.

The second argument against a loading dose is that patients beginning FIT are usually not in a state of absolute insulin deficiency, since they have been more or less reasonably controlled under conventional therapy.

Many patients have actually been using considerable amounts of long-acting insulins; for example, under common lente regimes, which use insulins that consist of 70% ultralente insulin. The effects of

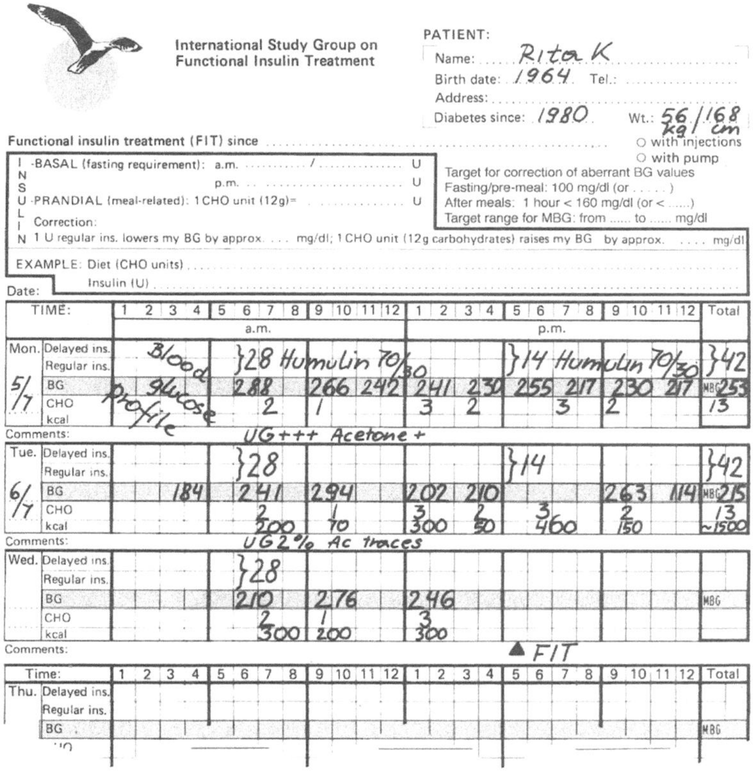
International Study Group on Functional Insulin Treatment

PATIENT:
Name: Rita K
Birth date: 1964 Tel.:
Address:
Diabetes since: 1980 Wt.: 56 kg / 168 cm

Functional insulin treatment (FIT) since
○ with injections
○ with pump

INSULIN
-BASAL (fasting requirement): a.m. / U
p.m. U
-PRANDIAL (meal-related): 1 CHO unit (12g)= U
Correction:
1 U regular ins. lowers my BG by approx. mg/dl; 1 CHO unit (12g carbohydrates) raises my BG by approx. mg/dl

Target for correction of aberrant BG values
Fasting/pre-meal: 100 mg/dl (or ......)
After meals: 1 hour < 160 mg/dl (or < ......)
Target range for MBG: from ...... to ...... mg/dl

EXAMPLE: Diet (CHO units)
Insulin (U)
Date:

TIME:		a.m. 1–4	a.m. 5–8	a.m. 9–12	p.m. 1–4	p.m. 5–8	p.m. 9–12	Total
Mon. 5/7	Delayed ins. / Regular ins.	Blood glucose profile	}28 Humulin 70/30			}14 Humulin 70/30		}42
	BG		288	266 242	241 230	255 217	230 217	MBG 253
	CHO		2	1	3 2	3	2	13
	kcal							
Comments:	UG+++ Acetone +							
Tue. 6/7	Delayed ins. / Regular ins.		}28			}14		}42
	BG	184	241	294	202 210		263 114	MBG 215
	CHO		2	1	3 2	3	2	13
	kcal		200	70	300 50	460	150	~1500
Comments:	UG 2% Ac traces							
Wed.	Delayed ins. / Regular ins.		}28					
	BG		210	276	246			MBG
	CHO		2	1	3			
	kcal		300	200	300			
Comments:						▲ FIT		
Thu.	Delayed ins. / Regular ins.							
	BG							MBG

Fig. 4.1. Example of algorithm generation.
A 22 year-old diabetic woman (Rita) learned the techniques of self-monitoring on Monday (parallel measurements with the training center's laboratory) and studied the various possibilities for insulin treatment on Tuesday. On Wednesday, she decided on multiple injections with a free diet. What algorithms (guidelines for insulin dosage) would you suggest for this patient?

Answer: Fasting insulin: ....

Prandial insulin: ....

Correction: 1 unit insulin ....
1 unit CHO ....

1. **Theoretical daily insulin requirement**
(modified from Waldhäusl et al. 1979)

Basal: (IU/24 h)	= (body wt in kg × 0.35)	56 × 0.35 =	20 IU/day
Prandial: (IU/day)	= (CHO units/day × 1.35)	13 × 1.35 =	18 IU/day
Total: (IU/day)			38 IU/day

2. **Estimating actual insulin requirement**
Under her current dose of 42 IU/day, the patient is ketotic, glucosuria is high, and her MBG is over 200 mg/dl. There is an insulin deficit. The actual insulin requirement can therefore be assumed to be about 10% higher than what she has been receiving (about 46 IU/day).

3. **Comparison of actual and theoretical insulin requirements (the quotient K):**

$$K = \frac{46}{38} = 1.21$$

4. **Creating algorithms (see also nomogram in Appendix 3)**

Basal insulin:	(0.35 × body wt in kg × K)		=
	0.35 × 56 × 1.21		= 23.71 IU/24 h
Prandial insulin	for 1 CHO unit:	(1.35 × K)	=
	(for 12 g CHO)	1.35 × 1.21	= 1.63 IU
	for 100 kcal protein/fat	(0.45 × K)	=
	(low-CHO meals only)	0.45 × 1.21	= 0.54 IU
Correction:	Change in BG (Delta BG) produced by		
Insulin:	1 IU = (−35 × 60/body wt in kg × 1/K)		=
	−35 × 60/56 × 1/1.21		= −31 mg/dl
Carbohydrates:	1 CHO unit = (+50 × 60/body wt in kg)		=
	(12 g CHO) +50 × 60/56		= + 53 mg/dl

5. **Rounding off the algorithms and handing over the working hypothesis to the patient:**
In our experience, slightly more insulin is needed to fulfill the basal requirement if delayed-acting insulin rather than CSII is used. Furthermore, approx. 10% of the total daily dose (4 IU) is added to the morning basal dose in the form of regular insulin (to compensate for increased early morning requirements). The following guidelines for insulin dosage are therefore given to the patient:

Basal: a.m.:	12 IU ultralente insulin (UL) + 4 IU regular (R)
p.m.:	12 IU ultralente insulin (UL)
Prandial:	1.6 IU per CHO unit (12 g CHO)
	(0.5 IU per 100 kcal noncarbohydrates-low CHO meals only)
Correction:	1 IU insulin lowers BG by −30 mg/dl (Delta BG)
	1 CHO unit raises BG by +50 mg/dl – " –

6. **Calculation of insulin dose (IU) for first day**
The patient plans to eat 4 meals consisting of 3 CHO units each:

Insulin:	12 UL 9 R	5 R	4 R	5 R 12 UL
CHO units:	3	3	3 (fruit)	3

This dosage would be correct as long as blood sugar remains within the target range. It should be written in the protocol as an example.

7. **Plausibility check:** The total insulin dose is 47 IU. The proportion of long-acting insulin is 24:47 = > 50%. The long acting insulin should therefore be reduced (e.g. to 11 IU in the evening).

N.B.:

(1) K illustrates the patient's insulin sensitivity for the physician! The patient needs concrete information rather than theoretical formulas! The information on K can be dispensed with for the patient. (See Chapter 8, "Rules for algorithm modification.")

(2) This patient's insulin regime during Phase I (just before the switch to functional insulin substitution) would no longer be typical today. Our current practice would be to change from the premixed insulin to separate injections of regular and delayed insulins (a "split and mixed regular plus NPH regime") before Phase 1.

these insulins can be expected to continue for some time after the change to FIT. So "loading" an already "loaded" patient would certainly not make sense.

4.4 Pedagogical Aspects of Insulin Substitution: Transactional Analysis and "Insulin Games"

Transactional analysis is a psychological theory which attempts to explain why people behave the way they do in understandable concepts (Berne 1961). What does this have to do with diabetes?

Successful functional insulin treatment presupposes active, blood glucose-contingent management of insulin administration by the patient for the rest of his life. This long-term process, like the treatment of other chronic diseases in which the active participation of the patient is required, functions optimally only when the patient has sufficiently attained the following:

(1) information (theoretical knowledge),
(2) applied knowledge, i.e. the necessary practical skills,
(3) motivation, and
(4) acceptance of his disease.

These four components determine the effectiveness of insulin substitution. There are a number of indications that diabetes education programs which affect only the patient's information status, and doubtfully at that, have no relevant effect on his metabolic situation and so hardly increase therapeutic efficiency (Worth et al. 1982). A method that is capable of influencing all four of these components will have a much greater chance of success. It is comparatively simple to produce improvements in theoretical knowledge and practical skills, but **how can one influence motivation and acceptance of diabetes, which are the final determinants of diabetes-related behaviors in the long run?**

The Teaching Letter of the Diabetes Education Study Group of the European Association for the Study of Diabetes (1985) put it this way: "Some overweight diabetic patients never lose weight despite consistent dietary advice. Some diabetic patients on insulin will not consistently test their urine or blood despite constant requests to do so. Some patients fail to carry sugar or sweets despite hypoglycemic episodes."

"These patients probably **could** learn, but they fail to **retain** or **integrate** important messages. These patients may **know** what they **should** do, but fail to do it."

"These are typical examples of lack of motivation to learn and to put learning into practice: they reflect a failure of the diabetes care team to successfully motivate the diabetic patient."

Transactional analysis (TA) is a useful tool for trying to understand and modify this kind of behavior. It was conceived as a method of examining social intercourse within a framework of psychotherapy by Eric Berne (1961) and systematically developed and described by Thomas A. Harris (1967) in the book *I'm OK – You're OK*, and by Amy and Thomas Harris in *Staying OK* (1985). TA is eminently suited to aid in understanding patient behavior, particularly in the field of diabetes care. It may not be fully accepted by the entire "psychological establishment," since it is a simple descriptive system that does not attempt to provide analytical explanations of causes. Its value, however, lies in its practicality, its willingness to do without technical jargon, and its ability to make complex psychological processes understandable to lay persons.

TA is based on the assumption, supported by observation, that coexisting in all human beings are three personality states. "It is as if in each person there is the same little person he was when he was three years old. There are also within him his own parents. These are recordings on the brain of actual experiences of internal and external events, the most significant of which happened during the first five years of life. There is a third state, different from these two. The first two are called Parent and Child, and the third, Adult" (Harris 1967).

In contrast to psychoanalysis, "Parent, Adult, and Child are not concepts like Superego, Ego, and Id...but phenomenological realities" (Berne 1961). Each "state is produced by the playback of recorded data of events in the past, involving real people, real places, real decisions, and real feelings" (Harris 1967). Through association, stimuli in the present can evoke the playback of this stored information, thus producing the corresponding ego state. The person thus responds to the present on the emotional level of whatever state has been produced.

Harris describes certain body and verbal clues that can help us to identify which ego state – the Parent, the Adult or the Child – happens to be in force at a given moment.

How can one tell that the **Parent** is in control? Physical clues include the furrowed brow, pursed lips, the pointing index finger, foot-tapping, sighing, etc. Verbal clues include words su ch as always, never, stupid, disgusting, naughty, revolting, ridiculous, dumb, etc.

How can the **Child** state be identified? By such physical clues as tears, pouting, temper tantrums, but also laughter and delight; or by verbal clues such as phrases like I want, I wish, I don't care, or superlatives such as bigger, biggest, best – as anexpression of the Child state's beloved game, "mine is better."

What characterizes the **Adult?** Openness, a listening attitude, and looking the partner in the eyes are examples of physical clues. Prime examples of verbal clues are rational questions: Wh y? What? Where? Who? How? How much? In what way? Or words such as probable, possible, unknown, objective, relative,and phrases such as I believe, I think, in my opinion, etc.

Transactional analysis can help us to understand interpersonal communication (transactions). Harris distinguishes between "complementary" transactions and "crossed" transactions.

In a complementary transaction each partner responds on alevel appropriate to the partner's current state. Either both respond on the same level, or each responds on the level being addressed by the other. Here are some examples of complementary transactions (Harris 1967).

Parent-Parent:

Lady 1: Kids nowadays are lazy.
Lady 2: It's a sign of the times.

Adult-Adult:
Stimulus: What time is it?
Reaction: I have 4:30.
Parent-Child:
Husband: I feel terrible.
Wife: Poor baby! Go lie down and I'll make you a cup of tea.

In crossed transactions, partners respond on the basis of their own "not OK" needs, rather than to what the partner is actually saying. In contrast to complementary transactions, crossed transactions lead to termination of the conversation. For example:

Patient (Adult addressing Adult): I'd like to work in a hospital like this.

Nurse (Parent addressing Child): You can't cope with your own problems (Harris 1967).

Doctor (Adult addressing Adult): I see your blood sugar levels have been high this week.

Patient (Child addressing Parent): I can't help it. I had two business dinners and on Sunday we had to eat at my mother-in-law's.

Now, how can transactional analysis help us reach our goals? If we use it not only for analyzing verbal communications, but also for a-nalyzing behavior, it can provide us with important knowledge regarding motivation.

In the analysis of our wishes and goals (Harris and Harris 1985), one should actually ask, "Which level of my personality wants this?" Take the case of an individual who wishes to write a book about the treatment of diabetes. Whether the book actually gets written or not seems to depend on *which state of the would-be author's personality* is operative. In the Parent state it is a comm and ("I must, I should"), while in the Child state it is a desire ("I want to"). It can be argued that the book will only be finished if the Child contributes the necessary motivation. If the wish is only on the Paren t level, the strong feeling that "I must" arouses anxiety in the Child. This may be enough to ensure a certain degree of motivation, but probably not for long. If the wish is solely on the Child level, however, it probably will not be written either, since the Child considers neither the consequences of an action nor other aspects of reality.

The Adult must also participate, since this state is the one responsible for the "how" of carrying out an action. Sometimes the Adult and

Child work together successfully, even if the Parent state does not cooperate ("I shouldn't, but I can and I want to"). When all three states cooperate ("I should, I can, I want to"), then a thing is most likely to actually get done. The desire on the part of the Child is in any case an absolute prerequisite for motivation.

In other words, in the therapy of a chronic disease the question of motivation can be reduced to the question of how to activate the patient's Child on a long-term basis. What does FIT ha ve to offer the Child? Freedom? Action? Accomplishment (i.e. lowering blood sugar)? The Child has no patience. It wants an instant solution, that works immediately. It wants to get rid of the high blood sugar right now. The Child also wants a sense of security ("If I can keep my blood sugar down, then I probably won't have to suffer late complications....") and of meaning ("... and since I can't be absolutely sure that I can prevent the late complications, at least I am not going to give up my quality of life!").

The Child must experience for itself that blood sugar can be actively raised or lowered, and that controlling it can be fun. The "insulin games" that are part of the FIT training program can be thought of, therefore, as nothing other than a dialogue between the trainer and the Child of the patient.

It is not hard to win the Adult over to FIT. That can be done by giving the patient sufficient factual information. The Adult will be responsible for choosing the type of therapy. But no amount of theoretical knowledge can guarantee good control if the Child does not cooperate.

How can we best mobilize the Parent for the purposes of FIT? Any opportunity to do something to improve one's health is likely to appeal to the Parent. If a patient's need to be "like everyone else" arises from the dictates of the Parent recording ("Don't do anything that's out of line!"), then the opportunity to behave "like a normal person" offered under FIT should satisfy the Parent. However this need to conform arises (it could also be a result of the need for security experienced in the Child state), we have found that helping to fulfill it is an extremely powerful motivational force, especially for younger patients.

The role of the Parent should not be underestimated, especially its potential for causing difficulties. The Parent is responsible for a bad conscience when blood sugar values are too high or too low. This is only of limited use, however, since guilt seldom leads to constructive

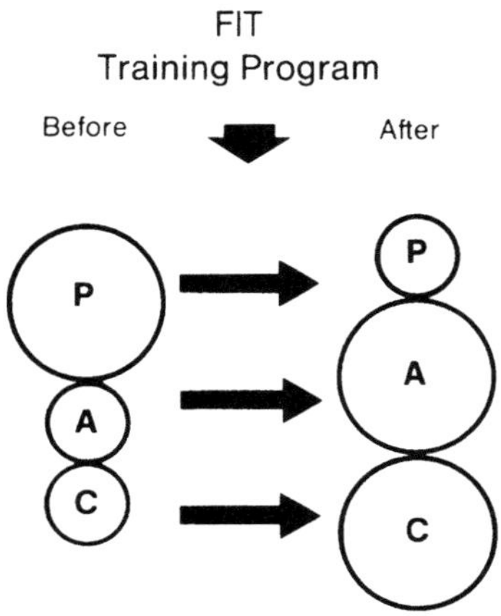

Fig. 4.2. FIT training from the standpoint of transactional analysis. **Before** the training program (under conventional therapy), a system of commands and prohibitions (P = Parent) is responsible for glycemic control (e.g., inject at ....., eat at ...., don't eat ...., etc.). **After** the training program, blood sugar level is controlled by means of acquired skills (A = Adult), supported by wishes (C = Child)

behavior. It would be much more sensible to activate the Adult in such situations, since analyzing the cause, immediate correction, and making plans for the future are done in the adult state. The Parent is also responsible for a patient's perfectionist inclinations. It is fine to try for the best, but poorly understood perfectionism can often lead to much too drastic corrections of hyperglycemia on the assumption that glycemic control has to be absolutely perfect.

Thus, when the training goals of functional insulin treatment are considered from the standpoint of transactional analysis, the following aspects are important. The wishes of the Child and the Adult are decisive for motivation, but all three components of personality can be utilized to manage the rehabilitation process (Fig. 4.2). The Child can be won over if it has the pleasure of being independent and active, and if its impatience can be satisfied with the possibility of immediate action. With its ingenuity, which is ultimately responsible for the success of FIT, and with its sense of humor as well, the Child can be of immense help in coping with problems.

The Adult is indispensable for processing the information necessary to evaluate the quality of the insulin substitution and for decision-making. Perhaps the value of the Parent lies in setting limits when the other two fail ("... I guess maybe I shouldn't eat that chocolate ..."), and being responsible for the necessary "oughts" and "shoulds" (keeping up the records, contact with the diabetes center, etc.). The Parent should not be allowed to become too powerful, however: **a bad conscience about hyperglycemia is useless. Perfectionism in diabetes control usually leads to problems.** Optim al control of type I (insulin-dependent) diabetes does not mean perfect metabolic control. Optimal control means achieving the highest quality of life and the best level of control that are possible at an acceptable level of exertion.

4.5 Is "Yielding to Temptation" All Bad?

Under conventional insulin therapy, diet is strictly regimented according to time of meals and type and amount of food. It would be a serious transgression to "yield to temptation" under conventional insulin therapy, i. e., to give in to an urge to eat something – usually a high-carbohydrate food – that is not allowed in the planned diet. In the FIT training program, however, "yielding to temptation" is an exercise which leads to a change in the patient's way of thinking and behaving towards food. It is not a license to behave irresponsibly, but rather a method of teaching responsible behavior in dealing with the practical aspects of insulin substitution under everyday conditions.

In this exercise patients receive an assignment to eat something that they have long wanted to eat, but never dared to. This is done at a time when they are away from the training center, but in the company of other members of the group. A prerequisite for the experiment is a certain amount of experience in determining insulin dosage on their own, so the exercise should not be carried out until at least the 2nd or 3rd day after the switch to FIT. During the exercise, the patient must determine both the size of the insulin dose and the shape of the curve of insulin absorption needed for the type of carbohydrate to be eaten. His decision influences not only the amount of insulin, but also the mode of injection and the interval between injecting and eating. (Details are given in Sect. 5.2, "Prandial insulin substitution. Problems in dosing regular insulin.")

The didactic goals of responsibly "yielding to temptation" are for the patient to:

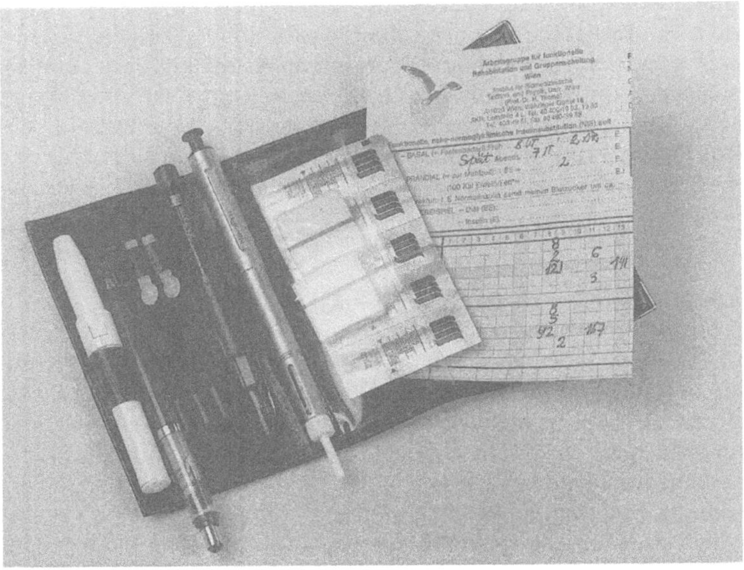

Fig. 4.3. The minimum equipment necessary for FIT ("mini-kit" to be carried at all times): blood glucose test strips for visual evaluation or a small blood glucose meter, regular insulin with an injection pen (or an insulin syringe), finger pricking device, glucose, log book. The figure shows an example of a pen-shaped glucose meter which allows rapid determination of blood glucose. Patients usually need not carry delayed-acting insulin with them during the day. (From: K. Howorka: Insulin-dependent? The functional use of insulin. Patient's handbook. Kirchheim, Mainz, 5th edition, 1995)

1. Test his ability to visually estimate the amount of carbohydrates in the foods he eats in a setting where weighing the food is not possible;
2. Test his ability to estimate his prandial insulin needs;
3. Test his ability to influence the course of postprandial insulinemia (by adapting the injection mode and the interval between injecting and eating to the type of meal consumed);
4. Test his ability to make adequate corrections of spontaneous blood glucose excursions;
5. Change his way of thinking about diet. Instead of thinking, "I'm not allowed to eat this," he learns to think, *"I can eat this if..."*;

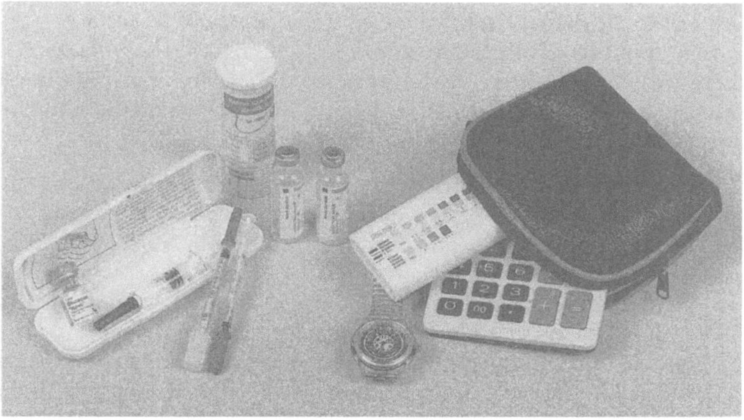

Fig. 4.4. Supplements to the FIT "mini-kit" (these items need not be carried at all times, but they should be readily accessible at home): Acetone and urine sugar test-strips, watch with s econd hand, insulin syringes, regular insulin in vials (even if the patient uses a pen, this is necessary in case of malfunction), delayed-acting insulin, glucagon, *blood glucose test strips to enable visual evaluation,* pocket calculator for calculating mean blood glucose. (From: K. Howorka: Insulin-dependent? The functional use of insulin. Patient's handbook. Kirchheim, Mainz, 5th edition, 1995.)

6. **Learn to recognize the limits of his ability to achieve normoglycemic insulin substitution;**
7. Test his ability to carry out insulin substitution when on his own (insulin administration, blood glucose estimation). Learn to assemble and check a "mini-kit" that should at least include regular insulin, blood glucose test strips, glucose, fixed-needle syringe and record sheet (see Fig. 4.3 and 4.4).

Points 5 and 6 are especially important. The other points can really be seen as a means for achieving these two. The ultimate goal of the exercise is a cognitive restructuring of the norms of the Parent and a transfer of responsibility to the Adult. Up to now, "yielding to temptation" has been "forbidden." From now on, the only thing that is "forbidden" is anything that the "data processor" of the Adult cannot handle, i.e., anything that cannot be rationally managed. In other words, if there are no rational reasons against an action, then it is allowed. Given proficiency in self-monitoring of blood sugar, adequate estimation of carbohydrate amount and type, and ability to adjust insulin accordingly, this leaves the diabetic patient a very great degree of freedom.

In order to avoid misunderstandings, I would like to emphasize that there are enough rational reasons against the routine consumption of rapidly absorbable carbohydrates to limit freedom where the eating of sweets is concerned:

(1) The amount of carbohydrates in such foods is very difficult to judge, so the risk of hyperglycemia or hypoglycemia is relatively great.
(2) The consumption of rapidly absorbable carbohydrates, especially by inexperienced patients, often leads to high postprandial blood glucose values. As previously mentioned, subcutaneous insulin administration is rarely able to achieve sufficiently rapid "postprandial" insulinemia. It is therefore necessary to use the various techniques available for speeding up insulin absorption (e.g., intramuscular administration, massaging of the injection site). Since a longer interval between injecting and eating is usually not practical, this problem might be most easily solved by using the fast-acting insulin analog that are currently being introduced (see Appendix 4). Experience with these preparations should allow evaluation of their clinical relevance in the near future.

The teaching goals of the "yielding" exercise that are mentioned in points 1–4 above refer to skills that are the province of the Adult: "Can I correctly and effectively carry out what I have learned?" One important reason for conducting this exercise during the training program in phase II of rehabilitation is that it gives the trainer an opportunity to check whether the patient is ready to take over responsibility for himself and to see how he handles it.

The following procedure for carrying out the exercise has been successful: Before an excursion away from the training center with other members of the group, the patients are instructed to eat and enjoy a special treat, something that they have dreamed of eating for a long time. They are asked to keep a written record of the experience and to ask themselves – in writing – the following questions:

- Can I choose the correct insulin dose for a given amount of carbohydrates?
- Can I choose the most suitable mode of insulin administration and the appropriate interval between injecting and eating?

- Have I got everything I need in my "mini-kit"? That is, am I equipped to correctly estimate my blood sugar (without a glucose meter) and to administer insulin when I am on my own?

The patients keep a running record of time, blood glucose (urine glucose is optional), physical activity, food consumed, insulin administered, etc., during the exercise. It is important to record everything, since without a written protocol it is impossible for either the trainer or the patient to analyze the experience. The results are discussed in detail on the next day.

We specifically recommend that the excursion be made only with other members of the group, unaccompanied by authority figures, i.e., anyone who would react on the "Parent" level in any interactions with members of the group (e.g., diabetes counselor, parents of teenage patients, spouses, etc.). When carried out within a group of patients undergoing the FIT training program, this procedure has an extremely positive effect on group dynamics.

4.6 Testing Algorithms for Correcting Blood Glucose (and Determining the Kidney Threshold for Glucose). Why?

In order to **test the validity of the algorithms for correcting off-target blood glucose values**, the patient first produces a controlled rise in blood sugar with oral glucose and later on a corresponding fall with regular insulin. If parallel measurements of blood and urine glucose are made at short intervals throughout the exercise, the patient's kidney threshold for glucose can also be determined. The exact procedure is shown in Fig. 4.5a,b.

This exercise is relatively laborious. Considerable fluid intake is of course necessary to ensure a sufficient quantity of urine. It takes hours, much patience on the part of both diabetic patient and trainer, and uses up numerous blood and urine glucose test strips. The question thus arises as to why it should be done at all.

The obvious reasons are that it can be useful to know at what level the kidney's threshold for glucose lies and how well the correction algorithms actually work:

- 1 carbohydrate unit (12 g) raises my blood sugar by ... mg/dl
- 1 unit of regular insulin lowers my blood sugar by ... mg/dl

Less obvious, but equally important goals of the kidney threshold exercise are didactic in nature:

- Comprehension of the relationship between glycemia and glucosuria;
- Understanding nature and limits of the predictability of blood sugar dynamics after carbohydrate or insulin administration;
- First hand experience of being able to actively influence blood glucose;
- Comprehension and acceptance of the fact that eliminating hyperglycemia takes a relatively long time, even if the mode of insulin administration is modified to facilitate absorption (e.g., even with intramuscular or intravenous administration).

Does this mean that in order to test the effect of regular insulin and/or oral glucose on blood sugar, all that is necessary is to administer regular insulin or glucose and observe the ensuing blood glucose dynamics? The answer is yes, as long as no other forces that might cause a relevant rise or fall in blood sugar are in effect during the test. In other words, it is necessary to achieve **basal conditions**, i.e., blood glucose stability, before one can test the validity of the correctionalgorithms and or determine the kidney threshold. As mentioned above, the second prerequisi te for this test is sufficient fluid intake. If the patient cannot produce enough urine, the test cannot be made.

Achieving basal conditions – simple in theory – is not easy at all in practice. In an insulin-deficient individual, basal conditions can theoretically be reached if the following conditions are achieved:

(1) Constant insulinemia
(2) Constant glucose production
(3) Stable and constant insulin sensitivity (which is representative of the patient's usual condition).

Constant insulinemia is reached when the actual insulin level is determined solely by a stable, nearly "linear" basal rate. The last injection of regular insulin – whether for compensation of food intake or correcting blood sugar excursions – should therefore have been made at least four hours previous to the beginning of the test.

Constant glucose production can be assumed if there is no relevant absorption of carbohydrates from the intestines, i.e. the last meal must have been consumed at least four hours previo usly. There should also be no loss of glucose through the urine. The patient's blood sugar should therefore lie below the kidney threshold at the beginning of the test. Hepatic glucose production also needs to be considered. For example, the patient should not fast on the day previous to the test, since hepatic glucose production may be reduced by decreased glycogen reserves. Optimally, patients should therefore maintain their usual diet (approx. 30 kcal per kg body weight) on the day before the test.

It is also important for **insulin sensitivity** to remain as constant (and characteristic) of the patient as possible during the test. Since most patients show circadian changes in insulin s ensitivity, with increased early-morning basal insulin requirements, mornings are not the best time to conduct the test. This means that the best time of day would generally be in the afternoon, about four hours after the noon meal.

Phase 1: Achieving Basal Conditions

During this phase, which takes several hours, a written protocol of the test is begun by patients and trainer working together (see Fig. 4.5 a,b). The questions to be answered are defined at the top of the form. Test procedure and technical requirements must be thoroughly discussed with the patients on the day before the test.

Three to four hours after the last meal, patients begin testing blood glucose every 30 minutes. It can be assumed that basal conditions have been reached when:

- there is no upward or downward trend in blood glucose,
- there is no glucosuria, and
- there is no ketonuria.

At the same time, the process of "hydration" must begin. Patients should drink at least one and a half to two liters (six to eight 8 oz. glasses) of calorie-free liquids. They should drink at least the first liter during this phase of trying to achieve basal conditions (about an hour before the beginning of the actual test). They can drink the second liter during the actual kidney threshold determination (phase 2).

Patient: Date: Trainer:

Technical requirements	Fulfilled: Yes	No
1. Glucose meter with adequate test strips available?	.....	.....
2. Acetone strips available?	.....	.....
3. Urine glucose test strips available?	.....	.....
4. Sufficient fluid available? (approx. 2000 ml, no beer, no milk, etc.)	.....	.....

In order to start the test, you need to be able to answer "yes" to all four questions. If not, please carry out the test another time when all the technical requirements can be fulfilled.

Phase 1: Fulfilling the prerequisites for kidney threshold determination. Achieving basal conditions.

	Yes	No
1. Last meal at least 4 hours ago?	.....	.....
2. Last regular insulin injection at least 4 hrs ago?	.....	.....
3. Blood sugar stable for last 1 1/2 hours? (No upward or downward trend.)	.....	.....
4. Urine sugar negative?	.....	.....
5. Urine acetone negative?	.....	.....

If you have answered "no" to more than one of these questions, the kidney threshold test will not give meaningful results. In this case you should conduct the test on another day when you are able to achieve basal conditions.
During Phase 1 you should drink at least 1 liter (four 8 oz. glasses) of any calorie-free liquid (water, mineral water, tea, etc.).

Phase 2: Controlled raising of blood glucose (Questions 1 and 2) Eat enough glucose to raise your blood sugar to about 250 mg/dl. Try to pass enough urine to measure urine sugar in 10-minute intervals. (This should be relatively easy if you have consumed at least 1 liter of fluid during Phase 1.) Measure your blood sugar at the same time that you measure your urine sugar. Drink another 1/4 to 1/2 liters (one to two more 8 oz. glasses).

Phase 3: "BG-Plateau"
Wait until your blood sugar has stabilized and does not drop spontaneously. Only then can you use your algorithms to calculate the amount of regular insulin you need to lower your blood sugar to about 100-110 mg/dl. Drink another 1/4 to 1/2 liters (one to two 8 oz. glasses).

Phase 4: Controlled lowering of blood sugar with regular insulin Inject the amount of regular insulin you have calculated will be necessary to lower your blood sugar to 100-110 mg/dl. In orde to save time, use the methods you have learned to speed up the action of regular insulin. Answer question 3. Continue to measure both urine and blood glucose in 15 minute intervals.

a

Fig. 4.5. Determining kidney threshold for glucose. **a** Patient instructions **b** Patient protocol

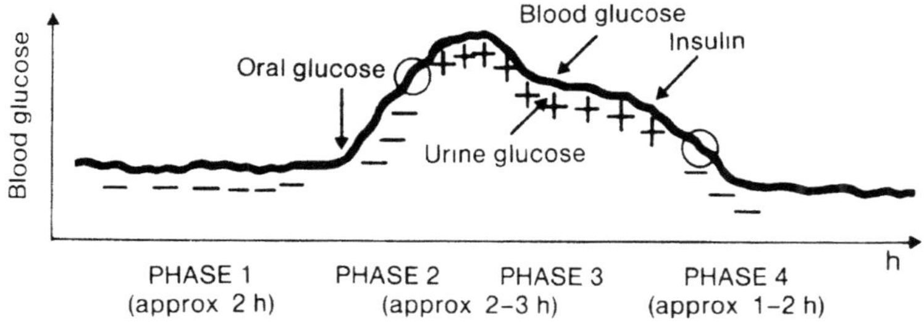

Questions: Under basal conditions

1. How high is my kidney threshold? .... mg/dl
2. What is the effect of 1 CHO unit (50 kcal) on my blood glucose? + ... mg/dl
3. What is the effect of 1 unit regular insulin on my blood glucose? – .... mg/dl

Time	Blood glucose mg/dl	+/– Urine glucose test strip	Action
Phase 1: Achieving basal conditions (approx. 2–3 h)			
....	....	....	Last meal at: .....
....	....	....	Last injection at: ..
....	....	....	Last correction at: .
....	....	....	with ....
....	....	....	because ....
Phase 2 + 3: Raising BG and reaching a BG-plateau (approx. 2–3 h)			
....	....	....	g glucose ....
....	....	....	....
....	....	....	....
....	....	....	....
Phase 4: **Controlled lowering of blood glucose (approx. 2 h)**			
....	....	....	IU regular insulin
....	....	....	....
....	....	....	....
....	....	....	....

Fig. 4.5b

On methodological grounds, the kidney threshold test can be divided into four phases:

(1) Achieving basal conditions;
(2) Controlled raising of blood glucose, determination of kidney threshold;
(3) Reaching a blood sugar plateau;
(4) Controlled lowering of blood glucose, testing of the algorithm, "One unit of regular insulin lowers my blood sugar by ... mg/dl."

Phase 2: Controlled Raising of Blood Sugar, Reaching the Kidney Threshold

Blood sugar is raised to a goal of about 240 mg/dl by means of controlled intake of oral glucose. This allows testing of the algorithm, "One carbohydrate unit raises my blood sugar by .... mg/dl." For example, assume that blood glucose has stabilized at about 110 mg/dl and is to be raised to 240 mg/dl. The initial algorithm is, "One carbohydrate unit raises my blood glucose by 50 mg/dl." In this case approx. 2.5 carbohydrate units should be consumed (approx. 30 g glucose) in order to test whether the algorithm is correct.

The kidney threshold is determined by simultaneous measurements of blood and urine glucose in approx. 10-minute intervals. Producing enough urine should be relatively easy if the patient has consumed at least one liter of fluids. The kidney threshold is defined as the blood glucose value at which glucose first appears in the urine.

Phase 3: Reaching a Blood Glucose Plateau

The patient must remember that it takes at least one hour to reach a blood glucose plateau after oral glucose intake. After a relatively steep rise, there is a spontaneous drop (due to distribution to other compartments), and finally a relative evening out to a plateau. The tendency to drop continues as long as the patient's blood sugar is above the kidney threshold. The **difference between the blood sugar level of the plateau and the value at the end of phase 1 (when basal conditions have been reached)** is the basis for testing the validity of the algorithm, "One carbohydrate unit raise my blood sugar by ... mg/dl."

Phase 4: Controlled Lowering of Blood Glucose

The algorithm, "One unit of regular insulin lowers my blood glucose by ... mg/dl," is tested by controlled administration of regular insulin. In order to save time, the patient can use the methods for speeding up insulin action which he will by this time have learned in the training program (see Sect. 5.2, "Prandial substitution. Problems in dosing regular insulin.") The required amount of insulin can be calculated from the difference between the blood glucose level of the plateau (phase 3) and the target value (usually 100 mg/dl). For example, if the initial algorithm assumes a drop in blood glucose of 40 mg/dl per unit insulin, and a plateau value of 220 mg/dl has been reached, 3units of regular insulin would be injected. If blood glucose is very high (plateau level above 250 mg/dl), then the probability of a further spontaneous fall due to loss of glucose through the urine must be taken into account. Here it would be advisable to make a "weaker" correction, i. e., to choose a somewhat higher target value, for example, 140 mg/dl, in order to avoid hypoglycemia.

After the administration of regular insulin, blood and urine sugar are again measured simultaneously, this time in intervals of about 15–20 minutes. The glucosuria does not disappear at the same level of blood sugar at which it appeared. This "hangover" effect is a good demonstration for the patient of the poor correlation between glucosuria and actual blood sugar.

The kidney threshold test requires a great deal of patience on the side of both diabetic patient and trainer. They must take into account that the entire procedure (including reaching basal conditions) takes about 5 hours. It must be made clear that it is not advisable to carry out the test unless:

- basal conditions can be achieved,
- the technical prerequisites can be fulfilled (see Fig. 4.5a),
- the didactic goals are attainable (a qualified trainer must be present),
- the necessary time can be spent.

The equipment to be used needs to be checked over before beginning the test. In order to avoid later problems with interpretation, each patient should measure blood glucose with the same instrument throughout the procedure. It is important to use sufficiently sensitive test strips for urine glucose. In order to demonstrate the lack of correlation between ketonuria and glucosuria, it is a good idea to also test for ketonuria.

It makes this somewhat complicated procedure more feasible and saves the trainer's time if patients are thoroughly instructed at the start and then left to carry out the test on their own. It is important, however, for the trainer to be available at regular 30–60 minute intervals for a few minutes in order to answer questions and help with interpretation.

Can it happen that the changes in blood glucose that are normally expected after administration of oral glucose or insulin do not occur? Could blood sugar remain high in spite of an injection of regular insulin, or fall in spite of carbohydrate intake? Such problems most frequently occur when true basal conditions have not been achieved, i. e., if there is either a state of relative hyperinsulinemia or hypoinsulinemia at the beginning of the test.

Hyperinsulinemia occurs either when the basal rate is too high or if too much regular insulin was administered at the last injection. A continuing fall in blood glucose, even a number of hours after administration of regular insulin, or a hypoglycemic episode during the first part of the test (during phase 1, when basal conditions are to be achieved), are indications that relative hyperinsulinemia exists. If hypoglycemia does occur, it should be compensated with 0.5–1.5 carbohydrate units (6–18 g) of oral glucose.

Relative hypoinsulinemia is usually the result of too little regular insulin having been injected before the last meal, or a basal rate that is too low. Indication's are prolonged hyperglycemia (even glucosuria) and a trend toward increasing blood glucose values. Theoretically, it might be possible in this case to conduct the kidney threshold test in reverse order, first lowering blood sugar, then raising it again. The predictive value of the test would suffer, however, particularly if there is glucosuria when the test begins. Unless basal conditions are reached, it is very difficult to verify the algorithms.

Finally, a word from the viewpoint of transactional analysis. It is **not** advisable to tell patients they **must** do something (consume glucose, inject insulin, etc.) Commands prevent positive response from the Child, and the real goal of the kidney threshold test is something that will ultimately be determined on the Child level. If the patient comes out of the experience with the conviction that:

I can deliberately lower my blood sugar, and
I can deliberately raise my blood sugar,

then the difficult kidney threshold test will be worth the effort. We should not forget that the patient can hardly "wish" (on the Child level) to actively manage his blood glucose unless he has **actually experienced** that it is relatively easy to do – if he uses the proper algorithms.

4.7 Why Fast?

How do you react to the suggestion that insulin-treated diabetic patients should fast? The idea runs counter to the prevailing norm that insulin-treated diabetic patients must eat regular meals – the same amount of carbohydrates every day.

Within the framework of the FIT training program, a one-day fast has nonetheless proved to be very useful as a means of testing the chosen method of basal insulin substitution, both in regard to dose and to the course of insulinemia over time. Testing the basal rate may be the obvious goal of the fasting exercise, but there are also other, more subtle goals.

Namely, fasting is the only way for patients to learn first-hand that with FIT, as long as only the basal component has been administered, it is not absolutely necessary to eat in order to prevent hypoglycemia. Again, this runs counter to the prevailing norm.

A further goal is for patients to grasp the fact that – even in a fasting condition – about 50% of the usual daily insulin dose is still necessary, or in other words, that insulin can never, under any circumstances, be completely omitted.

The fasting exercise also offers the opportunity for the patient to learn techniques for maintaining normoglycemic control under fasting conditions. This is very important in various situations that require a fasting state, such as surgery, gastroscopy, childbirth, etc.

One may well ask, "Who would want to fast, anyway?" Fasting should never be based on a "must" from the Parent. Would it not be better to appeal to the curiosity and need for independence of the Child? Given these incentives, we have found that almost all patients are willing to fast for one day. Indeed, many patients have told us afterwards that fasting – **instead of having to eat, finally to be allowed not to eat** – was practically the most important experience of the FIT training program. This illustrates the importance to patients of the change in norms under FIT, especially the liberation from being forced to eat.

The procedure for the fasting exercise involves doing without food for a total of about 36 hours. The last meal before fasting begins should be the evening meal, while the first meal after fasting ends should be breakfast on the day following the day of fasting. Patients measure their blood glucose as usual every 3–4 hours and correct any episodes of hypoglycemia or hyperglycemia on their own. Hyperglycemia is corrected with administration of regular insulin, and hypoglycemia with glucose intake (if blood glucose falls below 80 mg/dl). Blood glucose should be above 100 mg/dl at bedtime, just in case the basal insulin dose is too high.

What conclusions can be drawn from the day of fasting in regard to the basal insulin dose? If the patient needs to consume more than 2–3 carbohydrate units of glucose during the 36 hours because of low blood sugar values, then a reduction in the basal rate is advisable. Should several injections of regular insulin be necessary for correction of hyperglycemia during the 36-hour period, then a corresponding increase in basal insulin dose is recommended. The most important criterion for evaluating the basal insulin dose on the basis of the day of fasting is certainly not any one blood glucose value, but rather the net result of all corrections that were necessary during the fasting period. In this sense, it is also immaterial whether the patient starts the fasting day with normal or hyperglycemic values, as long as he immediately corrects his blood glucose to within his target range.

The importance of the day of fasting for evaluating the basal rate should not be overestimated, however. This exercise is only of limited value as a test of basal rate validity for the following reasons:

(1) Fasting during the FIT training program is usually done in a resting state, whereas under normal conditions, physical activity would lead to a decrease in basal insulin requirement.

(2) The best criterion of basal insulinization (see Sect. 5.1, "Basal substitution") is the stability of blood glucose under short-term fasting conditions, i.e., approx. 12 hours of fasting. Since the fasting exercise lasts considerably longer (36 hours), there will be a

reduction in glycogen reserves and a decrease in hepatic glucose production. We can assume that after about 20 hours of fasting the patient's usual basal insulin dose would be too high. Experience indicates that **the basal insulin dose is correct if the patient has to consume approximately 2 carbohydrate units (20–40 g) of glucose in order to prevent hypoglycemia during the fasting exercise.** For the same reasons, it is advisable to reduce the regular insulin component of the basal injection to about 50% of the usual dose.

5 Criteria for Functional Insulin Treatment

5.1 Basal Substitution

5.1.1 Basal Insulin

The basal insulin dose should ensure the stability of blood glucose during short-term periods of fasting. At present, the best method for replacing fasting insulin is probably continuous subcutaneous insulin infusion (CSII); however, a number of studies indicate that it is possible to achieve comparable levels of glycemic control using injections of delayed-acting insulins for basal insulinization (Rizza et al. 1980; Reeves et al. 1982; Schiffrin et al. 1982). As mentioned in Sect. 3.5.1, "Pharmacokinetics," insulins of the following types are suitable for substituting basal insulin with injections (the duration of relevant activity, which depends on dose, is given in parentheses): ultralente (18–30 h), lente (14–24 h), and NPH/isophane (10–18 h). With both CSII and injections, most patients need a small additional amount of regular insulin as a component of the morning basal dose in order to compensate for increased insulin requirements and prevent hyperglycemia after breakfast. This is usually around 10% of the total daily insulin requirement (i. e., 3–6 IU on average). Some patients also need a small supplementary dose of regular insulin in the afternoon or evening.

With injections, regardless of the type of insulin used, the basal dose should be administered twice daily in approximately equal amounts, usually after getting up in the morning and at bedtime. When injected twice daily, ultralente insulins have the advantage that the time point of the basal injection can be varied by up to 3 or 4 hours. For example, an ultralente insulin can be injected one day at 7 p. m. and the next at 10 p. m. With NPH and lente insulins, it is not advisable to inject in the early evening (e. g., before the evening meal), since their greater peak and shorter duration of activity might result in nighttime hypoglycemia and early-morning hyperglycemia.

Evaluating Dosage
Both patients and physicians should be able to judge whether the chosen dosage for basal insulin substitution is appropriate on the basis of the following criteria:

1. **Percentage of total daily insulin dose made up by delayed-acting insulin** under the patient's usual nutritional conditions;
2. **Stability of blood glucose during short periods of fasting,** e.g., overnight or between meals;
3. **Fasting blood glucose** levels.

1. Under the patient's usual dietary habits, the proportion of the total daily insulin dose made up by delayed-acting insulin is not less than 30% (35%) and not more than 50%.
2. It is important for the patient to choose a basal insulin dose that will maintain stable blood glucose levels during short periods of fasting. It must be emphasized that under FIT, fasting insulin should lead neither to a spontaneous fall nor to a spontaneous rise in blood glucose during an 8–10 h fast. In other words, **the basal insulin dose should ensure stability of blood glucose, although not necessarily normoglycemia.** Normoglycemia is achieved when the patient directly intervenes to correct blood glucose values that are out of the target range.
   During the day, numerous factors (meals, prandial insulin, exercise, etc.) influence the course of blood glucose. For this reason, it is simpler to use the short-term conditions of fasting overnight to evaluate the fit of basal substitution. As long as the interference of carbohydrates and/or regular insulin can be excluded, basal substitution can be considered to be correct if the blood glucose values at bedtime and at the probable nadir of blood glucose, i.e., at 3 or 4 a.m., are approximately equal. The difference between the nadir and the maximum of nighttime blood glucose, i.e., the difference between the values at about 3 a.m. and 7 a.m., should never be greater than 40 mg/dl.
3. In view of these considerations, it can be seen that the value of fasting blood glucose as a criterion for judging basal insulinization is only relative. Basal insulin should not lead to a fall in blood glucose, so if the patient is hyperglycemic when he goes to bed, he will still be hyperglycemic when he wakes up (if he made no corrections

at bedtime). If he is normoglycemic (within his target range) before he goes to bed, then his **fasting blood sugar should be above 90 and below 140 mg/dl.** A single fasting value outside of this target range does not mean that the basal rate should be changed, however. Such changes are made only when a trend is observed (see Chap. 8, "Rules for algorithm modification").

5.1.2 Fasting Hyperglycemia and Compensation of Circadian Variation in Insulin Requirements

The early-morning rise in blood glucose which occurs in diabetic patients was first described by Somogyi (1959) and named the "dawn phenomenon" by Maria Ines Schmidt (1979). The dawn phenomenon was more thoroughly investigated at the beginning of the 1980s (Bolli and Gerich 1984; Schmidt et al. 1981) and was shown to be a frequent problem for many patients. As a consequence of early-morning hyperglycemia, blood sugar levels are often elevated until almost noon.

It has also been shown that non-diabetic patients experience an early-morning increase in insulin requirement and corresponding increased insulin production (Schmidt et al. 1984). One cause of this phenomenon appears to be an increased production of growth hormone at the beginning of the night (Campbell et al. 1985).

In clinical practice, the dawn phenomenon seems to be a matter of a real physiological phenomenon that is often reinforced iatrogenically. Both inter- and intra- individual variability in the tendency towards early-morning hyperglycemia (Bolli 1984; Perriello et al. 1991) make therapeutic decisions sometimes difficult.

The following questions are important for type I diabetic patients under functional insulin treatment:

1. Does the rise in blood sugar usually occur before or after waking?
2. What is the course of blood sugar during the night?

1. Does blood sugar rise before or after waking?

If the tendency for blood sugar to rise occurs after 7 or 8 a.m., i.e., after waking, it is relatively easy to correct it with a small amount of regular insulin which is regarded as part of the basal rate. Another solution proposed by some investigators (Sonnenberg 1983) is to use a higher ratio of insulin per carbohydrate unit in the algorithm for prandial insulin for meals early in the day. A disadvantage of this solution is that it is complicated for the patient. He must remember to use different prandial algorithms at different times of the day. Furthermore, it forces him to eat breakfast in order to have high enough insulin levels to cover the morning. If he would like to postpone his breakfast, he will risk being hyperglycemic throughout the morning.

The problem is more difficult if the early-morning rise in blood glucose occurs before waking. Such elevated fasting values are indeed problematical for many patients. Before the basal insulin dose is modified, the following procedure should be followed (Table 5.1):

- The first thing to do is to verify that fasting values are indeed too high. A mean of fasting values under 140 mg/dl can certainly still be accepted in nonpregnant insulin-dependent patients. Delayed-acting insulins should be used sparingly.
- If early-morning hyperglycemia has been verified, then it is necessary to clarify whether the patient systematically corrects hyperglycemia at bedtime.
- It is also necessary to exclude the possibility of nighttime hypoglycemia, which could theoretically be followed by elevated blood glucose levels. (In this case the dosage of basal insulin must be reduced!) With low dosages of basal insulin, however, this posthypoglycemic hyperglycemia, also called the Somogyi effect (Somogyi 1959), is rare. Under FIT, if nighttime hypoglycemia does occur, then fasting values are also likely to be low. However, it is important to make sure that NPH or lente insulins were administered late, i.e., at bedtime, not before supper.

2. What is the shape of the blood glucose curve during the night?
When the above-mentioned factors have been investigated, the decision can be made either to change the shape of the basal insulin profile, or to globally increase the basal rate. The decision is made on the basis of the course of blood glucose during the night (see Table 5.1):

(a) **A constant rise in blood sugar throughout the night** without a low point at 3 or 4 a.m. indicates insufficient basal insulinization. The basal rate should be increased by about 10% a a first step. If an ultralente insulin is being used twice daily, then both the morning and evening doses should be increased. The reason for this is that, since such long-acting insulins have no distinct peak, given the circadian variations in fasting insulin requirements it is almost impossible to influence a circumscribed period of time. Other indications of a basal rate that is too low are a tendency to ketonuria and a low proportion (less than about 35%) of depot insulin as compared to total daily insulin dose.

(b) **If the nighttime blood glucose profile reaches a low point** at 3 or 4 a.m., then a global increase in basal rate is not advisable. If the patient went to bed with normoglycemic value s, an overall increase in the basal rate would probably produce hypoglycemia at 3 or 4 a.m. In this case it would be preferable to modify the shape of the basal insulin profile rather than to increase the overall basal rate.

If the patient has a programmable insulin pump, for example, he could set a higher alternative basal rate that would allow an increase during the early morning hours. Advocates of pump therapy therefore recommend using pumps with complex basal rates.

If the patient does not want a pump, the alternative would be a delayed-acting insulin with a distinct peak about 6 hours after injection, i.e., which would develop its maximum effect at about the time that insulin requirement increases. NPH and lente insulins have the desired characteristics (see Appendix 4). Administered at bedtime, these insulins would allow selective influencing of fasting blood glucose values. A morning injection of a long-acting insulin with a flatter profile (ultralente) would ensure a constant basal rate during the day. In the early morning, when insulin requirement is at its highest, both insulins would be available: ultralente from the previous morning's injection and NPH or lente from the late evening injection. This procedure also has the advantage that basal injection times are coupled to going to bed and getting up.

If for some reason a patient insists on using only one type of insulin for the basal rate, the following procedures might be tried:

- An NPH or lente insulin could be used for both morning and late evening basal injections. The shorter duration of action of these insulins might, however, lead to a period of relative insulin deficiency (a "hole") in the late afternoon and/or early evening, with a consequent need for corrections with regular insulin.
- The entire basal dose could be administered in one injection of an ultralente insulin in the evening. This has the disadvantage that there must be a fixed injection time, since even with ultralente insu-

International Study Group on Functional Insulin Treatment

PATIENT:
Name: *Peter G.*
Birth date: .... Tel.: ....
Address: ....
Diabetes since: *1980* Wt.: *70*

Functional insulin treatment (FIT) since ....

☒ with injections
○ with pump

INSULIN
- BASAL (fasting requirement): a.m. *15 UL / 3 REG* U
  p.m. *15 UL* U
- PRANDIAL (meal-related): 1 CHO unit (12 g) = *1,3 REG* U
- Correction:
  1 U regular ins. lowers my BG by approx. *-30* mg/dl; 1 CHO unit (12 g carbohydrates) raises my BG by approx. *50* mg/dl

Target for correction of aberrant BG values
Fasting/pre-meal: 100 mg/dl (or .....)
After meals: 1 hour < 160 mg/dl (or < ......)
Target range for MBG: from ...... to ...... mg/dl

EXAMPLE: Diet (CHO units) ....
Insulin (U) ....

Date:

TIME:		a.m. 1	2	3	4	5	6	7	8	9	10	11	12	p.m. 1	2	3	4	5	6	7	8	9	10	11	12	Total
Mon. 8/17	Delayed ins.	*ULTRALENTE*						15														15				30 / 54
	Regular ins.	*REGULAR*						12						8								4				24
	BG							210																	99	MBG 154
	CHO										3			6				2				3,5				~15
	kcal										400			600				150				500				~1900
Comments:																		*Football match*								
Tue. 8/18	Delayed ins.						15																	15		30 / 53
	Regular ins.						5					3		6					5					4		25
	BG						165										110						71			MBG 115
	CHO											2		4			1		2					3		12
	kcal											300		500			50		700					300		1800
Comments:																	*Jogging*									
Wed. 8/19	Delayed ins.								15														15			30 / 54
	Regular ins.								10				5							7			2			24
	BG								172														169			MBG 170
	CHO									4			3,5				1		5							~14
	kcal									400			600				50		800							~1800
Comments:																	*(H1)*									
Thu.	Delayed ins.							15																		
	Regular ins.							10																		
	BG							217																		MBG
	CHO																									
	kcal																									

Fig. 5.1. A normal-weight patient shows you this protocol. What would you advise him to do?

1. The diagnosis "high fasting BG values" is made.
2. Before modifying the basal rate, blood glucose should theoretically be measured at least once during the night, in order to exclude the possibility of nighttime hypoglycemia (which would indicate a reduction in basal rate), and to determine whether an intermediate insulin should be substituted for long-acting insulin in the evening basal injection, or whether both the morning and evening doses of long-acting insulin should be increased.
3. Since basal insulin already makes up more than 60% of the total daily insulin dose, the solution should be to change to an intermediate insulin (NPH or Lente-type – see Appendix 4). These insulins should be injected at bedtime, not earlier during the course of the evening.

Solution:

Previous basal rate:	a.m.:	15 IU ultralente + 3 IU regular
	p.m.:	15 IU ultralente
New basal rate:	a.m.:	15 IU ultralente + 3 IU regular
	(late) p.m.:	13–15 IU NPH

Comments:

The number of self-monitored blood glucose measurements is relatively low. Is the patient restricting himself to tests he can do with a glucose meter? If so, why? HbA_{1c}? As the combination of insulins for the basal rate is *much more effective* in controlling fasting values, it is advisable to reduce the dosage, at least initially.

Table 5.1. Procedure in case of high fasting blood glucose ("Dawn Phenomenon")

1. Are fasting values really too high? (Mean FBG greater than 140 mg/dl?)
2. Does the patient actually test blood glucose at bedtime and correct it if too high? Are fasting values still too high, even if the patient is normoglycemic at bedtime?
3. Can nighttime hypoglycemia (Somogyi effect) be excluded? (Blood sugar should be tested occasionally, i.e., once or twice a month, at about 3 a.m.)
4. What is the course of blood glucose during the night (when the influence of evening carbohydrate intake and/or regular insulin can be excluded)?

(a) Basal rate too low, no indication of increased early morning requirements

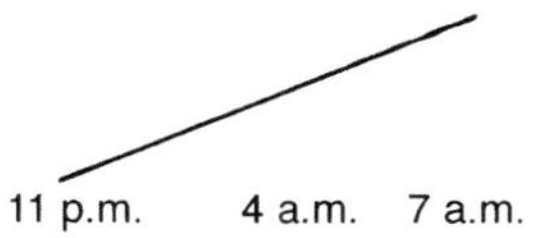

Increase basal rate "symmetrically": (the evening *and* the morning)

Limit: delayed-acting insulin should not make up more than 45–50% of total daily insulin requirement under normal diet (optimal proportion is 35–45%)

Other indices of too low basal rate:
Recurrent ketonuria.
Low ratio of delayed-acting insulin to total daily insulin.

(b) "True" increase in early morning insulin requirement

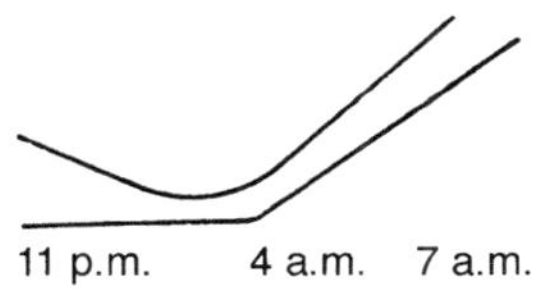

Modify shape of basal rate:

- NPH or lente insulin for late evening dose, + ultralente for morning dose

N.B.! Long-acting (ultralente) insulin **cannot** selectively influence **a circumscribed** period of the day in order to compensate for circadian variations in basal insulin requirements (e.g., the dawn phenomenon).

lins, there would not be enough basal insulin to cover requirements after 24 hours.

- The twice daily injections of ultralente insulin could be equally increased, as long as the patient agrees to consume an obligatory late-evening snack – without injecting prandial insulin – in order to avoid possible hypoglycemia during the night. This is not an ideal solution, however, since it is not really compatible with the principles of FIT, and it is somewhat risky. In any case, the amount of delayed-acting insulin should never be more than approximately half of the average daily requirement.

No advantages are given by 3 or 4 times daily application of delayed acting insulins (e.g. NPH insulin 4 times daily).

Summary
An increase in insulin requirements in the morning (and frequently also in the evening) does occur in an absolute majority of patients. This has also been demonstrated by data from patients with insulin infusion pumps with variable programmed basal infusion rates, which have been increasingly used in recent years. This is the also the reason why advocates of pump therapy recommend the use of pumps with complex basal rates.

When attempting to compensate for circadian variations in insulin requirements, it is relatively easy to produce a basal rate with multiple daily injections that is comparable to programmable CSII if the following strategies are used:

- **The use of NPH-insulin for the late evening basal injection,** while retaining ultralente insulin for the morning dose. This is the most important procedure for preventing the very frequent phenomenon of high fasting blood glucose (See Table 5.1)
- **Inclusion of regular insulin as part of the morning dose of basal insulin,** especially when the rise in blood glucose occurs after waking. This is to be considered a true component of the basal rate and is independent of prandial insulin for breakfast or any necessary blood glucose corrections. Occasionally, regular insulin is also included in the evening basal insulin dose.

In our experience, it is better to attempt to compensate for **circadian variations** in insulin requirement by means of the **basal rate** rather than by using different prandial/correct ing algorithms at different times of the day (e.g., more insulin per carbohydrate unit in the morning, and perhaps evening, than at midday). The simplicity of compensating for circadian variations by modifying the basal rate is particularly important when secondary adjustments of insulin dosage, i.e., algorithm modification to accommodate changes in total insulin requirements, are necessary (see Chap. 8, "Rules for algorithm modification").

The lower the dose of delayed-acting insulin used for basal insulinization, the stronger the circadian variations in insulin requirements – and the larger the amount of regular insulin required as a component of the basal dose (see Sect. 8.2.5, "Interdependence of algorithms").

5.2 Prandial Insulin Substitution – Problems in Dosing Regular Insulin

Under normal nutritional conditions, regular insulin makes up about 55–65% of the total daily insulin requirement. How should this insulin be distributed over the day? Prandial insulin should be administered whenever the patient eats. Since most people eat at least three meals per day, this works out to at least three injections of regular insulin per day. If more meals are eaten, it is possible **to cover two consecutive meals with one dose** (or one pump bolus), as long as the time interval between meals is shorter than 3 hours. Although this can be done (e.g., injecting enough regul ar insulin before a main meal to cover a planned snack later), it is not generally advisable under FIT. What if there is no time to eat the snack after all? In order to maintain maximum flexibility, it is better to inject before **each** meal. Whenever enough food is eaten to create a prandial insulin deficit of more than one to two units, insulin should be injected.

When injecting regular insulin, the patient must solve two related but separate problems:

(1) He must decide how much regular insulin to inject in order to cover the amount of food he plans to eat. **The appropriateness of the size of the chosen insulin dose can best be judged on the basis of late postprandial blood glucose values,** i.e., three to four (or even five) hours after the meal (or more exactly, after the injection).

(2) He must consider the dynamics of the course of postprandial insulinemia over time. The speed of insulin absorption needs to be adapted to the rate of carbohydrate absorption. **Early post pran-**

dial blood glucose values (i. e., 1-2 h) can be used to judge whether the level of insulin in the blood has risen quickly enough. In order to achieve adequate postprandial insulinemia, it is often necessary either to modify the usual subcutaneous mode of injection, slow down the absorption of carbohydrates, or lengthen the interval between injecting and eating (Lean et al. 1985).

The goal for the diabetic patient is to imitate the characteristics of prandial insulin secretion in healthy persons (immediate high insulinemia and direct hepatic effect of insulin produced by prehepatic insulin secretion), but this can be difficult in practice. One may smile at the techniques currently used for influencing the speed of insulin absorption. Nonetheless, it must be remembered that this is a problem that insulin-treated diabetic patients wrestle with several times a day, every day, since rapidly absorbable insulin analogs are still not available. The relevant fact is that regular insulin injected subcutaneously reaches its maximum activity only after approximately 1.5–2 hours, and (depending on size of dose) insulin activity usually ceases after 4–6 hours.

Yet in order to achieve an insulin activity profile comparable to that of non-diabetic persons, the **absorption of regular insulin should be accelerated** in any of the following situations:

(1) Consumption of carbohydrates, especially large amounts of rapidly absorbable carbohydrates;
(2) Correction of hyperglycemia;
(3) Compensation of circadian increases in basal insulin requirement by means of a component of regular insulin in the **morning** basal dose.

Under FIT there is really no other indication for using regular insulin, so that it is hardly an overstatement to say that **if regular insulin is to be used at all, it should act as quickly as possible!**

The following methods can be used to facilitate the absorption of regular insulin, thereby speeding up its action:
With subcutaneous injections:

- Production of local hyperemia by massaging the injection site (Berger et al. 1982)
- Local application of heat (Berger et al. 1982)

International Study Group on Functional Insulin Treatment

PATIENT:
Name: Irene L.
Birth date: 1953 Tel.:
Address:
Diabetes since: 1979 Wt.:

Functional insulin treatment (FIT) since .... ○ with injections ☒ with pump

INSULIN
- BASAL (fasting requirement): a.m. / p.m. } Σ 20U/24 h + 4U in the morning U
- PRANDIAL (meal-related): 1 CHO unit (12g) = 1,5 U
- Correction: 1 U regular ins. lowers my BG by approx. -40 mg/dl; 1 CHO unit (12g carbohydrates) raises my BG by approx. +50 mg/dl

Target for correction of aberrant BG values
Fasting/pre-meal: 100 mg/dl (or ......)
After meals: 1 hour < 160 mg/dl (or < ......)
Target range for MBG: from ...... to ...... mg/dl

EXAMPLE: Diet (CHO units) ....
Insulin (U) ....

Date:

TIME:		1 a.m.	2	3	4	5	6	7	8	9	10	11	12	1 p.m.	2	3	4	5	6	7	8	9	10	11	12	Total
Mon. 11/17	Delayed ins.									BASAL				RATE		20U/24h										
	Regular ins.								9																	
	BG								107		210			81												MBG
	CHO								3																	
	kcal								400																	
Comments:																										
Tue.	Delayed ins.																									
	Regular ins.																									
	BG																									MBG
	CHO																									
	kcal																									

Fig. 5.2. This patient is being treated with CSII
How would you interpret the course of blood sugar?
Is the insulin dose correct?

The suitability of the chosen regular insulin dose can best be evaluated on the basis of a late postprandial blood glucose value (3–5 hours after injecting or after a pump bolus). In this case the late postprandial value (just before lunch) was below the target range. The dose was about right, or perhaps a bit too high.

The value after breakfast does not allow any conclusions as to the correctness of the dose. A larger dose may have given better postprandial values, but would probably have resulted in hypoglycemia before lunch, unless a midmorning snack had been eaten.

The mistake was in the failure to achieve sufficient insulinemia immediately after eating. The interval between the bolus and the meal was too short (With injection therapy the patient would have had the alternative of facilitating insulin absorption; see Section 5.2).

- Muscle activity, increase of circulation time (Kemmer et al. 1980; other factors probably play a role here).
- Production of local hyperemia by means of salves (such as those used to combat rheumatic pain).

Change of injection mode:

- Intramuscular insulin administration
- Intravenous insulin administration (Schade et al. 1985).

The current introduction of fast-acting insulin analogs (see Appendix 4) inspires great hopes, since using insulin for correcting hyperglycemia or for covering prandial needs requires a much faster insulin effect than is possible with subcutaneous administration of **regular** insulin. The clinical usefulness of the fast-acting insulin analog Lispro (Humalog®) is currently being evaluated. In theory, that might be an ideal insulin for prandial and correctional purposes.

Of all present possibilities, only intramuscular insulin administration and the production of local hyperemia by massaging the injection site have become routine with our patients. Although we do not recommend injecting regular insulin intravenously, many of our patients have spontaneously used this route, usually when they want to quickly correct hyperglycemia before eating. No complications have yet resulted from this mode of administration. Patients claim that otherwise it remains relatively difficult to achieve a desirably high level of immediate postprandial insulinemia, at least after breakfast and/or when blood glucose is already elevated.

Instead of facilitating insulin action, another approach is to **slow down the rate of carbohydrate absorption.** Slowing the rate of carbohydrate absorption is indicated when postprandial insulinemia is inadequate, e.g., when there is hyperglycemia, and when carbohydrates are to be consumed either in large amounts or in a form that would otherwise be rapidly absorbed. Slowing carbohydrate absorption usually results in a decrease in postprandial insulin requirement.

Carbohydrate absorption can be slowed by the following measures:

- Decreasing the degree of processing or refining of carbohydrates (e.g., coarse instead of finely ground, raw instead of cooked, etc.), or using foods in which processing results in slow absorption (e.g., noodles).

- Increasing the proportion of non-carbohydrates in a meal, i.e., adding fat (Bernstein 1981; Chantelau et al. 1982). Beware of calories, however!
- Adding fiber or fiber-rich carbohydrates to a meal (raw vegetables, bran, legumes, "green" fruit with a high fructose content, commercial fiber-rich products, etc.).
- Adding gelatinizing substances.
- Reducing fluid intake during meals.
- Using absorption inhibitors such as biguanides or possibly alpha-glucosidase inhibitors (although there is still too little evidence to judge their worth).

In practice, a reduction in the carbohydrate content of an individual meal (with a corresponding increase in the noncarbohydrate content) is most effective in reducing postprandial hyperglycemia (Bernstein 1981; Chantelau 1982). However, in light of recommendations to reduce fat and increase the overall carbohydrate content of the diet, this strategy should not be encouraged for routine use. Another method of influencing postprandial insulinemia which has long been familiar, but relatively little used, is the **manipulation of the time period between injecting (or giving a pump bolus) and eating.** In order to assure an optimal blood glucose profile, this interval should be as long as possible (Lean et al. 1985; Dimitriadis and Gerich 1983), if no measures are taken to influence insulin kinetics. This solution is often impracticable, however. Not only is waiting irksome, but an unexpectedly delayed meal can cause havoc.

The interval between administration of regular insulin and eating should be at least 30 to 45 minutes, or even longer, in the following situations:

- Large meals with large amounts of carbohydrates;
- If the patient is hyperglycemic and decides he must eat (in this case, the interval should be several hours; or better yet, he should follow the rule, "If blood sugar is high, don't eat until you have corrected it");
- In the morning, when it is necessary to compensate for the "dawn phenomenon";
- When insulin is administered subcutaneously.

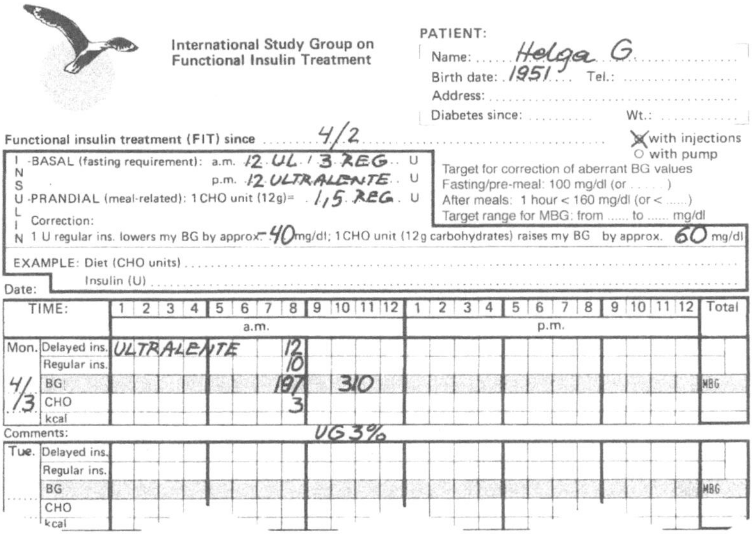

International Study Group on Functional Insulin Treatment

PATIENT:
Name: Helga G.
Birth date: 1951 Tel.:
Address:
Diabetes since: Wt.:

Functional insulin treatment (FIT) since 4/2

☒ with injections
○ with pump

INSULIN
- BASAL (fasting requirement): a.m. 12 UL / 3 REG U
  p.m. 12 ULTRALENTE U
- PRANDIAL (meal-related): 1 CHO unit (12g)= 1,5 REG U
- Correction:
  1 U regular ins. lowers my BG by approx. 40 mg/dl; 1 CHO unit (12 g carbohydrates) raises my BG by approx. 60 mg/dl

Target for correction of aberrant BG values
Fasting/pre-meal: 100 mg/dl (or ......)
After meals: 1 hour < 160 mg/dl (or < ......)
Target range for MBG: from ...... to ...... mg/dl

EXAMPLE: Diet (CHO units)
Insulin (U)
Date:

TIME:		1	2	3	4	5	6	7	8	9	10	11	12	1	2	3	4	5	6	7	8	9	10	11	12	Total
		a.m.												p.m.												
Mon. 4/3	Delayed ins.	ULTRALENTE							12																	
	Regular ins.								10																	
	BG								197		310															MBG
	CHO								3																	
	kcal																									

Comments: UG 3%

TIME:		1	2	3	4	5	6	7	8	9	10	11	12	1	2	3	4	5	6	7	8	9	10	11	12	Total
Tue.	Delayed ins.																									
	Regular ins.																									
	BG																									MBG
	CHO																									
	kcal																									

Fig. 5.3. This patient does not understand why her blood sugar was so high after breakfast, and does not know what to do.
How would you interpret it?
Did she choose the correct dose of insulin?
What should she do now? (It is 10:30 a. m.)

The patient ate breakfast in spite of considerable hyperglycemia. The further rise in blood glucose was to be expected.

If blood sugar is high, don't eat until you have corrected it!

Also discuss the interval between injecting and eating. Ask how she administered the insulin.

Since the hyperglycemia (310 mg/dl) was observed two hours after the meal, the dose of regular insulin must also have been too low.

Before correcting with another dose of regular insulin, the time period since the last correction must be considered. The interval should be at least three (or even four) hours. It is therefore better to wait about an hour before correcting, especially if the patient is at risk for hypoglycemia, since the last correction was made only two and a half hours ago.

Correct only to the target value (for 2 h pp: 140 mg/dl). The patient's blood sugar is too high by (310–140 =) 170 mg/dl. (Coulajshe have made a mistake in blood glucose measurement?) The correction can theoretically be made with (170:40 =) 4 units of regular insulin. Glucosuria is present, however. A part of the glucose will not "need" insulin to be transported, since it will land in the urine. The suitable dose would therefore probably be 3 IU.

How could she speed up the action of the regular insulin?

However, if insulin absorption is routinely speeded up (e.g., intramuscular injection) and no relevant hyperglycemia is present, we do not recommend this awkward solution and the interval can be relatively short.

The interval between insulin administration and eating can be especially short or even negative (injection after eating) in the following situations:

- Low carbohydrate meals;
- When insulin is administered intravenously (if blood glucose is relatively normal before eating, intravenous administration should only be carried out postprandially and only in exceptional situations). The dose should not be greater than 10% of the usual total daily requirement.

5.3 Self-monitoring and Glycemic Control – Why Keep Records?

A summary of the recommendations for blood glucose, urine glucose and acetone testing procedures under FIT was given in Table 3.1 (see Sect. 3.3, "Self-monitoring"). Both FIT and intensified insulin therapy usually require at least four self-monitored blood glucose measurements per day (Schiffrin and Belmonte 1982a) in order to maintain HbA_{1c} close to the upper limit of the normal range. Patients who have not been able to near-normalize HbA_{1c} should also be asked to test their urine for glucose. Namely, in such cases the problem is often that the patient is not making the necessary four blood sugar tests per day. He may be doing only three or fewer, usually because he cannot manage the practical problems involved.

Frequent self-monitoring alone does not guarantee good glycemic control, however. Numerous additional measures usually need to be undertaken by the patient in order to maintain his blood glucose levels within the desired range. The most important factor is therapeutic efficiency; in other words, the cost/benefit ratio in the maintenance of good metabolic control.

The following factors all play a role in achieving good glycemic control. Good record keeping in regard to these factors is therefore necessary in order to evaluate the success of therapy (see also Chap. 15, "Checklist for continuing care of FIT-patients"):

(1) Whether the patient keeps a record of self-monitoring, analyzes the data it contains each day, and makes decisions of the basis of the daily net result;
(2) Whether the patient can cope with the practical aspects of FIT;
(3) Frequency of acute complications;
(4) Whether the patient actually makes his insulin dose and carbohydrate intake contingent on blood glucose level.

5.3.1 Record Keeping, Analysis and Evaluation of the Daily Net Result

The physician cannot possibly evaluate therapeutic efficacy unless the patient brings him a written record. A special record sheet that allows a simultaneous overview of blood glucose values, insulin dose and food intake was developed specially for the FIT program. This record sheet is used in connection with objective laboratory data, particularly the HbA_{1c} value, in order to evaluate the effectiveness of therapy.

There are also other reasons for the patient to keep regular records. Good record keeping allows:

(1) An overview of the therapeutic decisions made by the patient;
(2) Prevention of mistakes in insulin administration due to forgetfulness;
(3) Recognition of recurring patterns in circadian variations of glycemic levels;
(4) Awareness of the frequency of hypoglycemic and hyperglycemic excursions.

The record should not contain only isolated numbers taken out of context, but should be an instrument that enables a daily "accounting." Almost the most important item is the daily total of insulin units administered. The sum of carbohydrate units and the total amount of calories consumed per day are also very useful (although counting calories is optional). The mean blood glucose (**MBG**) is a very good basis for judging the efficacy of glycemic control. It is a good idea for the patient to calculate the MBG at the end of each day (not practical without a pocket calculator). The MBG is only of real value, however, when at least 3–4 blood glucose tests are made each day and when at least one third of all measurements are random postprandial values.

The **weekly mean blood glucose** calculated from the daily MBGs is a very significant parameter of actual glycemic control. The weekly MBG should always be greater than 100 in non-pregnant patients (for patients with a high risk of severe hypoglycemia, greater than 120), but less than 160 (170) mg/dl. For "brittle," generally C-peptide negative patients who are active (e.g., working), but not influenced by any particularly strong motivational factors such as pregnancy, the weekly MBG usually lies between 120 and 160 mg/dl.

It is relatively easy to motivate most patients to carry out a daily "accounting" by calculating and comparing their daily total insulin (regular plus delayed-acting), carbohydrate consumption, and MBG (the latter with the help of a pocket calculator). The process takes no more than a minute. Of those patients who do keep good records, practically none show poor metabolic control. This is no epiphenomenon. **Patients trained in FIT learn to check and, if necessary, modify their algorithms for determining insulin dose whenever MBG falls below 100 (110) mg/dl or rises above 160 mg/dl on three consecutive days** (see Chap. 8, "Rules for algorithm modification").

The MBG also serves the role of a **"psychological buffer"** for especially ambitious and perfectionistic patients. Isolated blood glucose excursions need not be dramatized or overemphasized as long as the MBG is acceptable and no severe hypoglycemia occurs.

To be of value to the patient, the MBG must be calculated on a daily basis. Retrospective calculation "for the doctor" just before a clinic visit is as good as useless.

5.3.2 Coping with Practical Problems

Self-monitoring records can also help to identify deficits in practical knowledge and skills can stand in the way of good metabolic control. For example, correct substitution is impossible if the patient does not carry the proper equipment with him (insulin, syringe, dextrose and blood glucose test strips). **At any given time he must be able to ascertain his blood glucose level, evaluate it a nd, if necessary, correct it.** The inability to cope with the practical difficulties of insulin substitution usually is the result of either psychological factors (see Chap. 12, "Frequent patient- related problems") or, less frequently, lack of information. Psychological problems can and must be treated differently than simple lack of information.

5.3.3 Frequency of Acute Complications

All subjectively experienced feelings of hypoglycemia should be recorded and verified by means of a blood sugar test. These records can help to establish the frequency of perceived hypoglycemia. This frequency varies considerably in type I (insulin-dependent) diabetic patients, both intra- and inter- individually. The situation is similar for the occurrence of random blood glucose values under 50 mg/dl without perceived symptoms. Perception of hypoglycemia is important, since it is hardly possible to reach near-normal HbA_{1c} values without taking at least one or two mild hypoglycemic episodes per week into account (i.e., "H1" - see Chap. 6, "Hypoglycemia").

In analyzing the incidence of hyperglycemic excursions it is useful to be able to distinguish between moderate (approx. 240–400 mg/dl) and severe hyperglycemia (above 400 mg/dl – or out of range of a glucose meter). In the latter case it is important to test for acetone, since ketonuria can provide information as to the degree of the acute insulin deficiency. Further details are given in the chapters on hypoglycemia and hyperglycemia (Chap. 6 and Chap. 7).

5.3.4 Contingence of Insulin Dose and Carbohydrate Intake on Measured Blood Glucose Level

Adequate record keeping also helps to answer the following questions: Has the patient taken whatever action is necessary after every single blood glucose measurement? Does he actually correct all hyperglycemic values with insulin and all values below the target range (i.e., values below 80 mg/dl or, for patients at risk of severe hypoglycemia, under 90 mg/dl) with carbohydrate intake? Does he usually refrain from eating if he is hyperglycemic? Does he maintain appropriate time intervals between consecutive corrections of hyperglycemia with regular insulin? **It is particularly important to prevent "double corrections" of the same hyperglycemia.** The minimum time between two consecutive corrections of hyperglycemia with regular insulin should therefore be 3–4 hours.

What target level is chosen for corrections before a meal, for corrections after a meal? Targets of 100 (120) mg/dl for fasting and preprandial blood glucose and up to 160 (180) mg/dl for postprandial values are appropriate for about 80% of all patients. In special cases (e.g., patients with a high risk of hypoglycemia) the targets for correction of hyperglycemia and the target range for MBG should be individually selected (see Chap. 6, "Hypoglycemia").

In checking whether insulin dosage is contingent on glycemic levels, it is also important to consider whether the patient has made any modifications in insulin kinetics (see Sect. 5.2, "Prandial insulin substitution. Problems in dosing regular insulin"). We do not encourage using only subcutaneous administration with no modifications, but if the patient prefers to do so, then he must maintain an interval between injection and eating that is long enough – at least 30–45 minutes (Lean et al. 1985, Dimitriadis and Gerich 1983) – to provide for adequate levels of insulin, especially when a large meal is to be eaten.

6 Hypoglycemia

6.1 Definition of Hypoglycemia

Hypoglycemia has been defined (Berger et al. 1983a) as blood glucose below 40 mg/dl, or blood glucose below 50 mg/dl plus symptoms. In clinical practice, we find the condition that blood glucose must be below 50 mg/dl to be problematical, however, since up to 25% of patients already experience symptoms at around 60–70 mg/dl. Conversely, patients whose perception of symptoms is very poor often register blood glucose values between 40 and 50 mg/dl without symptoms, but which really should be classified as hypoglycemia. And self-prevention of mild hypoglycemia, which often occurs without symptoms during intensified insulin treatment, has a great importance in the re-establishment of the awareness of hypoglycemia (Cranston al. 1994; Fanelli et al. 1994; Howorka et al. 1996).

For practical purposes, it seems to us that the following modifications and division into types and stages can be helpful:

- H1 (mild hypoglycemia): either blood glucose under 60 mg/dl (capillary blood) with or without symptoms, or blood glucose under 70 mg/dl accompanied by symptoms, but with no relevant deleterious effect on rational behavior;
- H2 (moderate hypoglycemia): behavioral impairment due to hypoglycemia, but no unconsciousness;
- H3 (severe hypoglycemia): unconsciousness reported by patient, plus evidence of hypoglycemia as the cause;
- H4 (severe hypoglycemia and medical intervention): same as H3, but treated with glucagon or intravenous glucose administration.

This division is purely from a clinical point of view.

6.2 Increased Probability of Severe Hypoglycemia

Although hypoglycemia is still an unavoidable companion of insulin therapy, data on incidence, causes, possibilities for prevention and treatment under various therapy regimes and in particular patient groups have been surprisingly rudimentary up to now. It seems understandable that the long-term, near-normalization of blood glucose achieved by patient self-variation of insulin dose might carry a high risk of hypoglycemia. The following statements summarize clinical experience with the phenomenon of hypoglycemia.

In a typical diabetic population, the tendency towards hypoglycemia tends to cluster in certain high-risk groups. Although the mean frequency of hy poglycemic episodes in the total population may be low, a few individuals typically suffer considerably more frequent and more severe episodes than the average. Functional, near-normoglycemic insulin substitution can only be successful if all possible preventive measures are taken to keep the frequency of hypoglycemic episodes low, not only in the average patient, but especially in such high-risk groups. Thus, the FIT training program needs to pay special attention to both patient characteristics and types of situations that increase the risk of hypoglycemia in order to take the necessary therapeutic steps.

The characteristics of high-risk patients are summarized in Table 6.1. In addition to these patient characteristics, one can identify certain situations which increase the probability of hypoglycemia (for example, through failure to recognize symptoms). These are summarized in Table 6.2. The simultaneous occurrence of high-risk characteristics and high-risk situations seems to cause a nearly exponential increase in the probability of hypoglycemia.

Table 6.1. Characteristics of patients at risk for severe hypoglycemia

- History of severe hypoglycemia with unconsciousness
- "Type A behavior pattern," perfectionism, unrealistic glycemic goals
- Diabetes of long duration
- Low body mass index (underweight)
- Renal insufficiency
- Erratic insulin absorption kinetics due to lipohypertrophy and/or lipatrophy

Table 6.2. Characteristics of situations that increase the risk of hypoglycemia

- Overfatigue
- Alcohol consumption
- Restriction of food intake
- 1st and 2nd trimester of pregnancy
- Use of beta blockers
- Use of sympathomimetics
- Amphetamine and/or coffee consumption
- Certain psychological problems
- Failure to self-monitor
- "Blind" corrections of unverified hyperglycemia (!)
- Consumption of foods with unknown carbohydrate content (sweets)
- Physical activity without corresponding changes in carbohydrate consumption and/or insulin dose
- Inadequate patient education: errors in primary or secondary adaptation of insulin dosage; incorrect algorithms, e.g., basal rate too high (allows eating without rise in BG)
- Inappropriate counseling from physician or trainer (e.g., target value too low, etc.)

The risk arises either because there is a relative overdose of insulin, or because symptoms of hypoglycemia are not recognized.

6.3 Causes of Hypoglycemia

Under FIT, where all decisions regarding diet and insulin dose are made by the patient, the following causes of hypoglycemia are relevant:

1. Inaccurate dosage of prandial insulin – overestimation of carbohydrate amount;
2. Repeated correction of the "same" hyperglycemic excursion; too short a time interval between successive corrections of hyperglycemia. This is often a compounding error after the patient has already made the mistake of eating in spite of having high blood glucose levels.
3. Falsely defined blood glucose target (e.g., 80 mg/dl). Postprandial corrections with regular insulin are risky. Due to the relatively unpredictable absorption kinetics of both carbohydrates and insulin, they are especially hard to gauge. For this reason, the 1 h postprandial target level should be 160–180 mg/dl for correction of hyperglycemia.

4. Failure to correct below-target blood sugar values that were symptom-free, for example, values between 60–90 mg/dl.
5. Failure to consume additional carbohydrates to compensate for physical activity.
6. Erratic absorption kinetics of insulin, for example, if regular and delayed-acting insulins are mixed, or if there is lipodystrophy at the injection site.
7. Erratic absorption kinetics of carbohydrates.
8. Inappropriate algorithms for prandial insulin.
9. Inappropriate algorithms for correction of hyperglycemia.
10. Inappropriate dosage of basal insulin (basal rate too high). This occurs particularly often when intensively treated patients without proper FIT training try to vary their food intake. They often forget that they also need to take reduced food intake into account. Since the basic insulin requirement not only rises with increased food intake, but also drops when decreased food intake lowers hepatic glucose production, hypoglycemia will occur if the amount of basal insulin is not lowered correspondingly.

6.4 Prevention of Hypoglycemia

Particularly in the group of patients who experience frequent severe hypoglycemia, all possible steps should be taken in order to prevent hypoglycemia. One particular characteristic shared by many of these patients is their relatively poor ability to perceive hypoglycemia (White et al. 1983). This is often the result of impaired early counter-regulation (glucagon and catecholamine secretion). Symptoms such as sweating, shivering, etc., do not appear; the most prominent symptoms are rather those of the central nervous system (behavioral deficits). The awareness of hypoglycemia can nonetheless be improved by training. When blood glucose decreases to 40 or 50 mg/dl, many patients experience a particular, individually characteristic symptom; for example, a specific emotion such as anxiety or depression, which has no apparent cause. Others experience changes in perception; for example, of colors or patterns. When patients are trained to be particularly sensitive to these idiosyncratic signals and to **determine blood glucose level immediately**, a dramatic improvement in perception of hypoglycemia can be achieved.

Study groups of Stephanie Amiel (Cranston et al. 1994) and Bolli (Fanelli et al. 1993, 1994) showed that hypoglycemia per se leads to a worsening of the awareness of hypoglycemia, and that systematic prevention of hypoglycemia has a fundamental significance in improving the awareness of hypoglycemia. Hypoglycemia with loss of consciousness (White et al. 1983; DCCT Research Group 1991, 1993) high predictive value for increased risk of further serious hypoglycemia. The tendency to have serious hypoglycemia during intensified insulin treatment is also associated with certain behavioral characteristics such as a willingness to take the risks involved in accepting low blood glucose values. Such patients experience even short-term periods of blood glucose values above 200 mg/dl as catastrophic events and choose inappropriately low targets for their mean blood glucose; e.g., these patients often aim for mean blood glucose values under 120 mg/dl and HbA_{1c} values well within the normal range. For this reason, the targets for the control of glycemia are discussed thoroughly in the actual FIT training. Except for pregnant women, who should aim for lower values, the target HbA1c value should generally be at the upper limit of the normal range or even up to 1.5% over the upper limit of the normal range.

Experience shows that even this approach is not sufficient to restrain the before-mentioned "hypoglycemia risk group." We therefore started special group training sessions for people with a particularly high risk of hypoglycemia (two evenings). Our preliminary results show that only this specific, intensive training motivates patients with unrealistic glycemia targets to reduce their attempts to achieve almost normal glycemia, and to accept the principle of hypoglycemia prevention as the main step towards improving hypoglycemia awareness (Table 6.3).

We were, additionally, able to show that a remarkably high level of vigilance – even under basal conditions – is particularly characteristic of EEG results in patients with a history of hypoglycemia with loss of consciousness (Howorka et al. 1995).

Vigilance levels are inversely proportional to actual blood glucose levels, however: even mild hypoglycemia is accompanied by vigilance reduction in this group of patients. It was previously shown that a fall in blood glucose below 50 mg/dl is detrimental to intellectual performance (Holmes et al. 1983; Pramming et al. 1986). In some patients, except for this transient deficit, no other symptoms are discernible.

Table 6.3. Hypoglycemia and hypoglycemia unawareness
Contents of a group training program for patients with severe hypoglycemia

1. Normoglycemia versus hypoglycemia: terminology, physiology, "counterregulation" in nondiabetic and diabetic persons.
2. Characteristics of hypoglycemia unawareness: Frequency, behavioral features, high risk patients, high risk situations.
3. Formal pathogenesis: Hormonal and EEG response to hypoglycemia in patients with reduced hypoglycemia awareness or with a history of severe hypoglycemia.
4. Causal pathogenesis: Causes of the development of hypoglycemia unawareness.
5. Potential reversal of hypoglycemia unawareness: Hypoglycemia prevention – meaning, possibilities, procedures, hypoglycemia awareness training.
6. Individual evaluation of risk of hypoglycemia, working out personal measures to take, redefinition of personal therapy targets (work in small groups).

Even these patients are able to train themselves to detect their condition by means of an "intellectual barrier sensor." At the slightest suspicion of hypoglycemia, they make a habit of performing some relatively complex intellectual task; for example, multiplying 12 by 16 in their head – or reciting a poem or a childhood prayer – and timing their performance. If they are temporarily unable to perform the task, or if it takes twice as long as usual, they know that this could be an indication of otherwise symptom-free hypoglycemia. In the high-risk patient group the following axiom has proven helpful: **"If the world should suddenly seem different to you** – differently colored or patterned, or darker, or more complex – **then think first of the possibility of hypoglycemia."** Thus, training plays a considerable role in the improvement of hypoglycemia perception in the high-risk group.

It is also very important for the patient to be able to verify and correct mild hypoglycemia immediately, i.e., he must carry blood glucose test strips and some form of oral glucose with him at all times. Blood glucose values around 60 mg/dl should immediately be corrected to the target range of 90–100 mg/dl.

In the interests of preventing hypoglycemia, it is also important to adhere to the principle: **no more insulin than necessary.** This is particularly true for basal insulinization; hypoglyce mia should never be produced by the delayed-acting insulin. Therefore, the dosage of delayed-acting insulin should be kept as low as possible. For patients with a very high insulin requirement (over 80 or 90 units of insulin per

24 h with normal diet), it is useful to cover basal requirements with a combination of delayed-acting and regular insulins. In order to keep the amount of delayed-acting insulin as low as possible, it might even be advisable in such cases to accept slightly elevated fasting blood glucose values, as long as the mean is around 140 mg/dl.

The rule "no more insulin than necessary" applies to prandial insulin dosage as well. Although in principle it is possible to cover two consecutive meals with one injection of regular insulin, we recommend injecting before each meal in order to avoid a condition of hyperinsulinemia. This considerably reduces the risk of severe hypoglycemia; if he only has to worry about one meal at a time, the patient can better calculate exactly what and when he is going to eat.

Corrections of hyperglycemic excursions with regular insulin should also be guided by the same rule. Here it is important to consider the target range. If a correction is made postprandially, the target should not be below 160 mg/dl. The interval between successive corrections should be greater than 3–4 hours. If the value to be corrected is very high, the possibility of renal glucose loss must also be taken into account; a portion of the glucose does not "need" insulin for transport, since it is excreted by the kidneys. It is therefore advisable to make a "weak" correction if blood glucose is around or above 300 mg/dl, i.e., to choose a target of about 140–160 mg/dl, even if the correction is for a preprandial value. In this way, the spontaneous drop in blood glucose due to glucosuria can be taken into account.

It may also be advisable to generally raise the blood glucose target for correction of hyperglycemia in high-risk patients; for example, to 120 mg/dl preprandially, up to 200 mg/dl postprandially. An alternative would be for the patient to modify his algorithm for correcting blood glucose. If his algorithm assumes, for example, that one unit of insulin produces a fall in blood sugar of 40 mg/dl, he could modify it to assume a fall of 50 mg/dl. There is a well-known rule of thumb (Bernstein 1981) that "one unit of regular insulin decreases blood glucose by 30 mg/dl." This is in fact not true for most patients who have an insulin requirement of under 45 IU/day. To say that one unit of insulin produces a 40 mg/dl drop would be more generally correct. For the hypoglycemia risk group, increasing the target value and increasing the algorithms for the reduction of blood glucose by one unit of regular insulin rank among the most important principles of avoiding hypoglycemia during functional insulin treatment (see Appendix 3).

Most **situations with a high risk of hypoglycemia** arise when more than the usual number of "stress factors" impinge on the patient, causing him to fail to recognize symptoms. This situatio may interact with certain personality characteristics, leading to a tendency to overdose insulin. In high-stress situations, patients also tend to make fewer blood glucose determinations than usual, compounding the problem. In situations that increase the risk of hpoglycemia, the rule should be, "make more, not fewer blood sugar tests!"

In situations involving greater responsibility (e.g., school examinations, long drives, etc.), a kind of "controlled hyperglycemia" might even be advisable. While such situations last, the preprandial target range could be purposely raised, for example, to about 130 mg/dl. It would not be advisable, or even feasible, to raise the preprandial target above 140 mg/dl, however. At these levels considerable swings in blood glucose arise, partly from the impossibility of maintaining "basal conditions" above the kidney threshold. We recommend that the preprandial blood glucose target for patients with a high risk of hypoglycemia or for high-risk situations should be set at about 110 mg/dl (up to a maximum of 140 mg/dl). This would correspond to a realizable target range for mean blood glucose (MBG) of 130–160 (170) mg/dl.

A last comment concerning the prevention of hypoglycemia. The concept of near-normoglycemia is often associated with the fear of hypoglycemia. However, the differentiation of insulin dosage according to required function makes FIT per se a very efficient means of preventing severe hypoglycemia. The distribution of insulin over a number of small portions, each contingent on blood sugar level, is a most effective protection against hypoglycemic episodes. FIT successfully avoids the hazardous hyperinsulinemia which is a constant companion of conventional insulin therapy, forcing patients to eat 6–7 times a day.

We have often been confronted with the claim that conventional therapy protects against hypoglycemia. It must be emphasized that a twice-daily dose of insulin, with the resulting pre-programming of the necessity for numerous meals, is logically much more dangerous. The greater the individual's risk of hypoglycemia, the more important it is that insulin should be administered in a directed, differentiated and function-contingent (i.e., FIT-compatible) form. Under both conventional and intensified insulin therapy, many patients undergo numerous episodes of unconsciousness in spite of self-monitoring and dietary discipline, without even achieving normal HbA_{1c} levels. But after switching to FIT, these patients often experience only a negligible frequency of hypoglycemic episodes and are able to achieve (near) normal levels of glycosylated hemoglobin, in spite of a fully flexible diet and sometimes even fewer self-monitored blood glucose tests than before. It is absolutely necessary for such patients to utilize all the above-mentioned techniques for hypoglycemia prevention including the mentioned hypoglycemia group training, however, in order to achieve this therapeutic success.

6.5 Treatment of Hypoglycemia

Even under FIT, it is practically impossible to achieve good metabolic control without at least some episodes of mild hypoglycemia, although not all patients will experience severe hypoglycemia. It is thus very important for every patient to know what to do in case of hypoglycemia.

The treatment of mild (often symptomless) hypoglycemia consists of the **immediate intake** of rapidly absorbable carbohydrates (oral glucose). Approximate ly 6–12 g are usually sufficient (more rarely, up to 20 g). Fluid intake facilitates intestinal absorption. Foods containing **fats or protein are not suitable** for treating hypoglycemia, since carbohydrate absorption is slowed.

The aid of another person is required if there is a behavioral deficit (H2) or if the patient has lost consciousness (H3). Glucose can be administered buccally after it has been moistened, but glucagon is the treatment of choice if the patient is unconscious (1 mg; either s.c., i.m. or i.v. administration). Glucagon can now be considered standard treatment for severe hypoglycemia with unconsciousness. Therefore, **every insulin-treated diabetic person should have glucagon in his home. Proper instruction of persons living in the same household** is an absolutely necessary component of every insulin therapy. After the glucagon has been administered and the patient has regained consciousness, one or two carbohydrate units should be eaten in order to prevent a renewed drop in blood glucose. In rare cases where the liver contains no glycogen reserves, the administration of glucagon will not be effective. If such is the case, glucose must be administered intravenously.

International Study Group on Functional Insulin Treatment

PATIENT:
Name: *Thomas H.*
Birth date: .... Tel.: ....
Address: ....
Diabetes since: *1970* Wt.: ....

Functional insulin treatment (FIT) since .... ○ with injections ○ with pump

INSULIN
- BASAL (fasting requirement): a.m. *13 UL / 4 REG* U
  p.m. *13 UL* U
- PRANDIAL (meal-related): 1 CHO unit (12g)= *1,3 REG* U
- Correction:
  1 U regular ins. lowers my BG by approx. *-30* mg/dl; 1 CHO unit (12g carbohydrates) raises my BG by approx. ..... mg/dl

Target for correction of aberrant BG values
Fasting/pre-meal: 100 mg/dl (or .....)
After meals: 1 hour < 160 mg/dl (or < ......)
Target range for MBG: from ...... to ...... mg/dl

EXAMPLE: Diet (CHO units) ....
Insulin (U) ....
Date:

Day	TIME:	1 a.m.	2	3	4	5	6	7	8	9	10	11	12	1 p.m.	2	3	4	5	6	7	8	9	10	11	12	Total
Mon. 2/27	Delayed ins.	*Ultralente*							*13*													*13*				*26*
	Regular ins.	*Reg.*							*10*			*5*		*10*						*2*		*10*				*37* *63*
	BG								*140*					*108*						*140*						MBG
	CHO								*4*			*3*		*~7*									*~4*			*~18*
	kcal									*600*		*400*		*450*									*500*			
Comments:																										
Tue.	Delayed ins.			*Glucagon!*																						
	Regular ins.																									
	BG			*(H4)*																						MBG
	CHO																									
	kcal																									
Comments:																										
Wed.	Delayed ins.																									
	Regular ins.																									
	BG																									MBG
	CHO																									
	kcal																									

Fig. 6.1 The patient (a 23 year-old medical student) had a severe hypoglycemic attack yesterday that required outside help (glucagon injected by his girlfriend). What questions would you ask?
What action would you suggest?

1. According to the case history the patient has the following high-risk characteristics for hypoglycemia:
1.1 H3 (How often?)
1.2 Ambitious – medical student
1.3 Long duration of diabetes (over 15 years)
1.4 Lipohypertrophy
1.5 Frequent high risk situations – coffee drinker, internship, examinations coming up

2. Make sure patient is aware of high-risk characteristics and situations

3. Prevention
3.1 Raise blood glucose target (to approx. 110–130 mg/dl) and change correcting algorithm from: "1 IU regular insulin lowers my blood glucose by approx. –30 mg/dl" to "... by approx. –40 mg/dl").
3.2 Avoid high-risk situations. Do not inject into areas with lipodystrophy!
3.3 Check other algorithms for insulin dosage. (Evidently the patient injected much more regular insulin than was necessary. Try to uncover the actual cause. Although the hypoglycemia only occurred at 4 a.m., the problem seems to be the evening dose of regular insulin, not the delayed acting insulin.)
3.4 Does the patient have glucose (dextrose) handy at all times?
3.5 What about testing blood glucose at bedtime?
3.6 Considering his hypoglycemia risk profile, this patient does not test blood glucose often enough.
3.7 Prescribe new package of glucagon.
3.8 Invite the patient to attend group training for hypoglycemia prevention (Table 6.3).

If there are no other complications, hospitalization is not necessary, neither during nor after a severe hypoglycemic episode. In fact, it could even do more harm than good. **Instead of hospitalizing a patient, the following is advisable:**

(1) Immediate treatment of the hypoglycemia (H3)
(2) Rest and proper food
(3) Analysis and discussion with patient of causes, plus mapping out a strategy for future prevention

The three steps outlined above usually take a maximum of about one hour. Dramatization of the situation is pointless. Both severe hypoglycemia and repeated mild hypoglycemic episodes are occasions for evaluating and, if necessary, modifying the algorithms for insulin dosage.

7 Hyperglycemia

Blood glucose values above 160 mg/dl (or to be more exact, any value above the set target range) are defined as hyperglycemic under FIT.

The following factors may cause hyperglycemia in patients under FIT (listed in order of clinical importance and without consideration of psychological problems):

1. Underestimation of the speed of carbohydrate absorption; i.e., too short an interval between injecting and eating (with subcutaneous insulin administration). Underestimating the speed of carbohydrate absorption results in only a **short period of postprandial hyperglycemia.**
2. Underestimation of the amount of carbohydrates. This problem can often be recognized on the basis of fact that the **resulting hyperglycemia is prolonged** over several hours.
3. Fasting hyperglycemia (dawn phenomenon) – inadequate basal insulinization.
4. Infections, acute illnesses, etc., that lead to an acute, global increase of insulin requirement; for example, infection with fever.
5. Using inappropriate algorithms for dosing prandial insulin.
6. Reactive hyperglycemia following hypoglycemia, i.e., the "Somogyi effect" (Somogyi 1959). This is very rare under FIT, however, even in cases of erratic, short-term insulin overdoses.
7. Errors in arithmetic when using algorithms to calculate insulin dose.

The treatment of hyperglycemia under FIT involves a **primary adjustment** of insulin dose, i.e., a **blood glucose correction** using the algorithm, "one unit of insulin reduces my blood glucose by ... mg/dl." Thus, any hyperglycemic valuecalls for an immediate reaction in the form of an injection of regular (soluble) insulin with the goal of lowering blood glucose to the target level. The only exception is an interval since the last correction of less than 3–4 hours. In order to shorten the period of hyperglycemia, no food could be eaten until blood sugar is again within the target range.

The underestimation of carbohydrate absorption and amount (points 1 and 2) are the the most frequent causes of hyperglycemia under FIT. They do not call for a modification of the algorithms for insulin dosage, rather only for correction of the current hyperglycemia.

If several successive acute corrections of hyperglycemia are necessary, i.e., if insulin requirement is increased and/or insulin dosage is insufficient due to infection (point 4), incorrect algorithms (point 5), or possibly the dawn phenomenon (point 3), then not only should the immediate hyperglycemic value be corrected, but the algorithms need to be modified as well. The **modification of algorithms** is called a **secondary adjustment of insulin dosage.** The following chapter presents detailed guidelines for algorithm modification.

8 Rules for Algorithm Modification

With the algorithms, "One unit of regular insulin lowers my blood sugar by ... mg/dl," and "One carbohydrate unit raises my blood sugar by ... mg/dl," patients can immediately correct any blood glucose value that is off-target. Experience shows that patients do indeed have no trouble making such primary adjustments of off-target blood glucose values. It is much more difficult to learn make secondary adjustments of insulin dosage, i.e., to independently adjust the algorithms (the underlying rules for basal and prandial insulin and for correcting off-target values). Nevertheless, in addition to acute correction of blood glucose, the algorithms occasionally do need to be adapted or revised.

In changing the insulin dosage algorithms (i.e., making secondary adjustments), two problem areas should be differentiated:

(1) There may be a global change (either increase or decrease) in insulin sensitivity (as measured by insulin requirement), so that the algorithms for basal and prandial insulin as well as for correcting off-target values need to be adapted to accommodate the new conditions.
(2) A particular algorithm (whether for basal or prandial insulin or for corrections) may not be adequate and must therefore be revised.

8.1 Global Changes in Insulin Requirement

In practice, the patient can only identify changes in insulin sensitivity on the basis of changes in his daily insulin requirement or level of glycemic control (MBG). Proficiency in keeping and analyzing daily records of blood glucose, amount of insulin administered, and

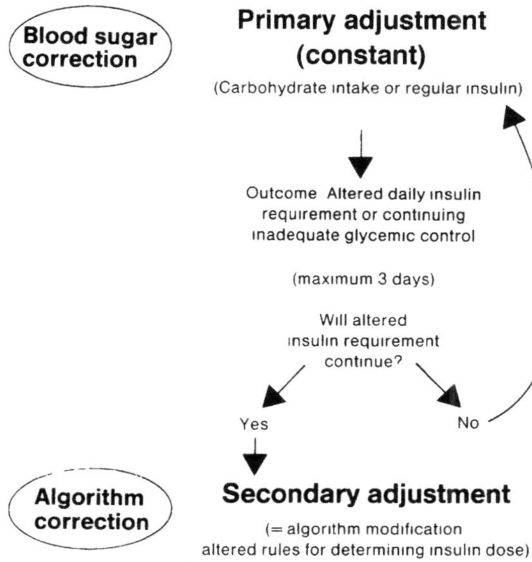

Fig. 8.1. Primary and secondary adjustments of insulin dosage made by FIT patients.

amount of food consumed each day is absolutely necessary in order to alter algorithms efficiently. **Without balancing these factors against each other, algorithm correction would be impossible, since the patient would not be able to correctly estimate his daily insulin requirement.**

A **primary adjustment** involves correcting blood glucose with either regular insulin (for hyperglycemia) or carbohydrates (for hypoglycemia). Primary adjustments are "perpetual"; they are necessary again and again, whenever blood glucose values are outside the target range (see Fig. 8.1).

If the patient recognizes a persisting change in insulin requirement, he makes a **secondary adjustment** of insulin dosage by modifying his algorithms in proportion to changes in mean daily insulin requirement.

As a rule of thumb, to obtain the new values, the algorithms for basal and prandial insulin can be multiplied by the quotient:

$$\frac{\text{current daily insulin requirement (IU)}}{\text{mean previous daily insulin requirement (IU)}}$$

An analogous modification in the algorithm for determining the reduction in blood glucose produced by one unit of regular insulin can be made using the following equation:

$$\begin{array}{l}\text{New difference value}\\ \text{(Delta BG per unit}\\ \text{regular insulin)}\end{array} = \begin{array}{l}\text{Value of}\\ \text{previous}\\ \text{algorithm}\end{array} \times \frac{\begin{array}{l}\text{mean previous daily}\\ \text{insulin requirement (IU)}\end{array}}{\begin{array}{l}\text{current daily insulin}\\ \text{requirement (IU)}\end{array}}$$

The fit of the secondary adjustment then must be tested on the basis of further self-monitoring and analysis of blood glucose levels in comparison to insulin dosage and food intake.

8.1.1 Global Decrease in Insulin Requirement

A global decrease in insulin requirement, i.e., amount of insulin administered, means a reduction in K (see Sect. 4.1, "Initial Algorithms, 'K' and the Blood Glucose Target Value"). Such decreases can be caused by a number of factors, including increased physical activity (see Chap. 9, "Physical Activity"), reduced food intake, cessation of chronic stress and/or illness, conclusion of puberty, termination of pregnancy (birth), renal insufficiency, and relative normalization of blood glucose after a period of hyperglycemia with a resulting improvement in insulin sensitivity.

Excessive insulinization due to a global reduction in insulin requirement can usually be recognized on the basis of an increased frequency of hypoglycemic episodes or a decrease in MBG to below 100 mg/dl (under 110 mg/dl for patients with a high risk of hypoglycemia) for three consecutive days. If there is an increased frequency of hypoglycemia, other causes such as errors in dosing prandial insulin must be excluded before the algorithms are modified (see Chap. 6, "Hypoglycemia").

An increased frequency of hypoglycemia or a lowered MBG should invariably cause the patient to consider whether a secondary adjustment of the algorithms is necessary. He will have been making primary adjustments (corrections of current blood glucose), which in practice means either increasing carbohydrate intake or omitting part of the dose of regular insulin. If ongoing evaluation makes it clear that

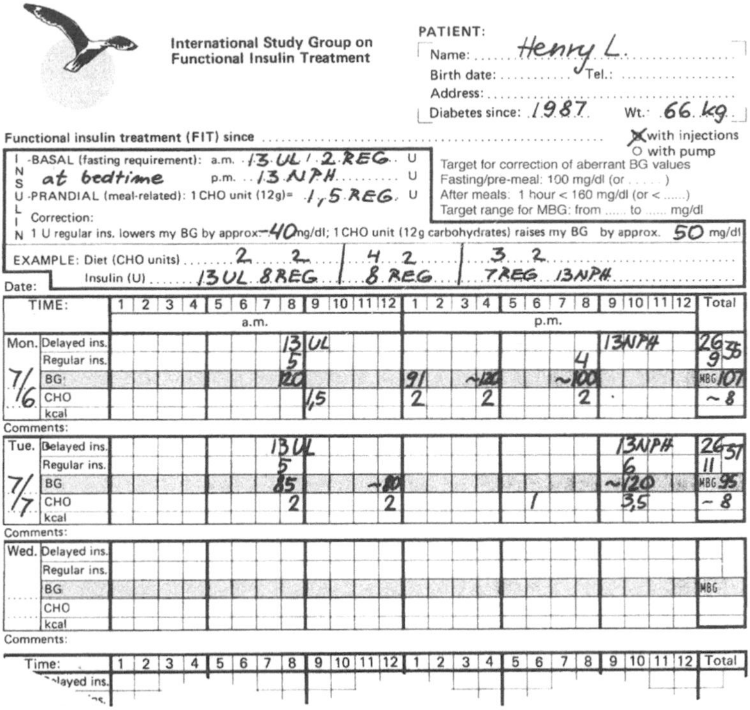

International Study Group on Functional Insulin Treatment

PATIENT:
Name: Henry L.
Birth date: .... Tel.: ....
Address: ....
Diabetes since: 1987 Wt.: 66 kg

Functional insulin treatment (FIT) since .... ☒ with injections ○ with pump

INSULIN
- BASAL (fasting requirement): a.m. 13 UL / 2 REG U
  at bedtime p.m. 13 NPH .... U
- PRANDIAL (meal-related): 1 CHO unit (12g) = 1,5 REG U
- Correction:
  1 U regular ins. lowers my BG by approx. 40 mg/dl; 1 CHO unit (12 g carbohydrates) raises my BG by approx. 50 mg/dl

Target for correction of aberrant BG values
Fasting/pre-meal: 100 mg/dl (or ......)
After meals: 1 hour < 160 mg/dl (or < ......)
Target range for MBG: from ...... to ...... mg/dl

EXAMPLE: Diet (CHO units) 2 2 | 4 2 | 3 2
Insulin (U) 13UL 8REG | 8 REG | 7REG 13NPH

Date:

TIME:		a.m. 1	2	3	4	5	6	7	8	9	10	11	12	p.m. 1	2	3	4	5	6	7	8	9	10	11	12	Total
Mon. 7/6	Delayed ins.								13 UL													13NPH				26 (35)
	Regular ins.								5												4					9
	BG								120					91			~120				~100					MBG 107
	CHO									1,5				2			2				2					~8
	kcal																									

Comments:

TIME:		a.m. 1	2	3	4	5	6	7	8	9	10	11	12	p.m. 1	2	3	4	5	6	7	8	9	10	11	12	Total
Tue. 7/7	Delayed ins.								13 UL													13NPH				26 (37)
	Regular ins.								5														6			11
	BG								85				~80									~120				MBG 95
	CHO								2				2						1				3,5			~8
	kcal																									

Comments:

TIME:		a.m. 1	2	3	4	5	6	7	8	9	10	11	12	p.m. 1	2	3	4	5	6	7	8	9	10	11	12	Total
Wed.	Delayed ins.																									
	Regular ins.																									
	BG																									MBG
	CHO																									
	kcal																									

Comments:

Time:	1	2	3	4	5	6	7	8	9	10	11	12	1	2	3	4	5	6	7	8	9	10	11	12	Total
Delayed ins.																									

Fig. 8.2. A 35-year-old office worker completed the FIT training program two months previously and brings the following diary to his first follow-up visit. What questions would you ask?
What recommendations would you make?

The long-acting insulin component of the total daily insulin dose is 70-75%, which suggests that the basal rate is too high. The reason for omitting the midday dose needs to be clarified. Apparently with this regime the patient can- and must-eat "to keep up with the basal rate," i.e., food intake does not lead to a rise in blood sugar, even when the dose of short-acting insulin is omitted.

Clearly the original dosage scheme (see "Example of therapy") is no longer valid. The current insulin requirement is about 35 IU, not 50, as was previously the case, but the patient has neglected to make the necessary secondary adjustment (algorithm correction).

The patient (normal to underweight) should also be asked why he eats so few carbohydrates (8 CHO units per day, which corresponds to only 400 kcal from carbohydrates). It can be assumed that his diet is high in fat.

Summary:

1. Reduce basal insulin (to approx. 9 – 9 ultralente)
2. Inject regular insulin for midday meal
3. Make sure patient knows how to make secondary adjustments in insulin dosage (algorithm modification)!
4. Consume more carbohydrates. (Optional: note caloric intake to clarify the amount of noncarbohydrate nutrients.)

there is indeed a change in daily insulin requirement, the patient must ask himself the following question before making the secondary adjustment (i.e., before modifying his algorithms): Will the change in insulin requirement (insulin sensitivity) continue? If the answer is yes – for example, in the case of an extended skiing vacation, after giving birth, or renal insufficiency, etc. – then the algorithms should be changed. If the change is only temporary, for example, if strenuous physical activity is planned for only one day, then a primary adjustment is sufficient without changing the algorithms.

8.1.2 Global Increase in Insulin Requirement

An overall rise in daily insulin requirement, i.e., an increase in insulin resistance as expressed by the quotient K, is most often caused by acute illness, especially if fever is present. It can be the result of other factors such as weight gain, pregnancy, etc., as well.

Insufficient global insulinization is indicated by persistent hyperglycemia (mean blood glucose above 160 (170) mg/dl on at least three successive days), if other causes of hyperglycemia such as carelessness or underestimation of amount of carbohydrates consumed (see Chap. 7, "Hyperglycemia") have been excluded. Inadequate insulin dosage is also signaled by excessive increases in the regular insulin component of total daily insulin (i.e., increase in corrections necessary to keep blood glucose within target range), or the presence of ketonuria (and/ or glucosuria).

The steps taken by the patient to control blood sugar under conditions of increasing insulin requirement are analogous to those for decreasing requirement. Primary adjustments are based on correcting off-target values with regular insulin. It is necessary to observe the rule, "Eat only after correcting hyperglycemia," if normal blood sugar levels are to be restored quickly.

Once the new daily insulin requirement has been estimated, the patient must decide whether the new conditions will continue for some time (e.g., in the case of a broken leg, pregnancy, etc.), or whether they will be short-lived (e.g., fever returning to normal, etc.). If the patient thinks they will continue, then he carries out the secondary adjustment (modifies the algorithms). If he thinks they will be short-lived, he will only take care of the situation by continuing to make primary adjustments (correcting off-target blood sugar values).

8.2 Modification of Individual Algorithms

Modification of a single algorithm should be carried out when there are particular recurring problems with glycemic control, but no certain indication of a global change in insulin requirement.

Even when optimal algorithms are being used, both hypoglycemia and hyperglycemia can still occur (see Chap. 6, "Hypoglycemia," and Chap. 7, "Hyperglycemia"). The most frequent cause is inaccurate estimation of carbohydrate content and/or absorption rate of food. The algorithms should therefore **not** be changed as long as the cause of deviant blood glucose values is in doubt.

From the beginning of FIT on, the patient should be expected to:(a) make autonomous suggestions regarding the adjustment of algorithms; (b) refuse to take suggestions for algorithm modification, unless rational and understandable reasons are given; and (c) make any modifications to single algorithms only in steps of 10–20%, at most.

8.2.1 Modifying the Algorithm for Basal Insulin

The following signals indicate that basal insulinization is inadequate and the basal rate should be increased (by 10% as a first step):

- Elevated fasting blood glucose (See Sect. 5.1, "Basal Substitution");
- Low proportion of delayed-acting insulin to total daily insulin (i.e., under about 35%);
- Recurrent ketonuria and spontaneous BG-increases.

Excessive basal insulinization (and the need for a reduction in delayed-acting insulin) is indicated by the following situations:

- Spontaneous fall in blood glucose overnight during at least two consecutive nights;
- Relatively low fasting blood glucose (60–90 mg/dl);
- High proportion of delayed-acting insulin in the total daily insulin dose (over 50%);
- The patient can – and must – "eat to keep up with the basal rate" (he is normoglycemic in spite of food intake without prandial insulin), without this being due to increased physical activity;
- Weight loss or commencement of a reducing diet. After even a few

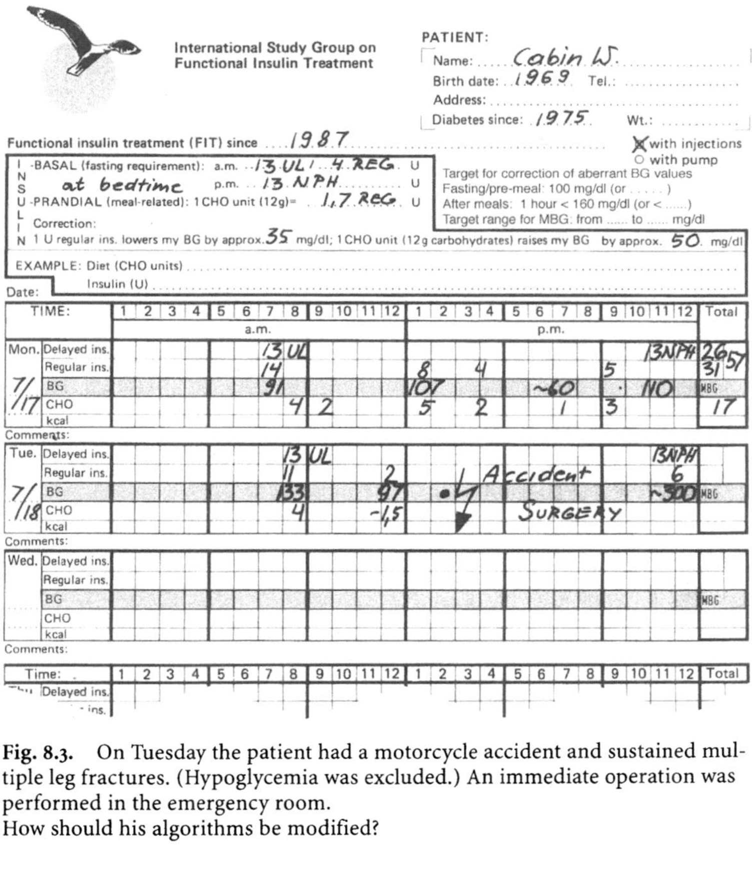

International Study Group on Functional Insulin Treatment

PATIENT:
Name: Cabin W.
Birth date: 1969 Tel.:
Address:
Diabetes since: 1975 Wt.:

Functional insulin treatment (FIT) since 1987 ☒ with injections ○ with pump

INSULIN -BASAL (fasting requirement): a.m. 13 UL / 4 REG U; at bedtime p.m. 13 NPH U
-PRANDIAL (meal-related): 1 CHO unit (12g)= 1,7 REG U
Correction: 1 U regular ins. lowers my BG by approx. 35 mg/dl; 1 CHO unit (12g carbohydrates) raises my BG by approx. 50 mg/dl

Target for correction of aberrant BG values
Fasting/pre-meal: 100 mg/dl (or .....)
After meals: 1 hour < 160 mg/dl (or < ......)
Target range for MBG: from ...... to ...... mg/dl

EXAMPLE: Diet (CHO units)
Insulin (U)
Date:

TIME:		a.m. 1	2	3	4	5	6	7	8	9	10	11	12	p.m. 1	2	3	4	5	6	7	8	9	10	11	12	Total
Mon.	Delayed ins.							13 UL																13NPH		26
	Regular ins.							14						8			4					5				31 57
7/17	BG							91						107						~60				NO		MBG
	CHO								4	2				5			2			1		3				17
	kcal																									
Comments:																										
Tue.	Delayed ins.							13 UL																13NPH		
	Regular ins.							11					2				Accident							6		
7/18	BG							133					97			• ↯								~300		MBG
	CHO								4				-1,5					Surgery								
	kcal																									
Comments:																										
Wed.	Delayed ins.																									
	Regular ins.																									
	BG																									MBG
	CHO																									
	kcal																									
Comments:																										

Fig. 8.3. On Tuesday the patient had a motorcycle accident and sustained multiple leg fractures. (Hypoglycemia was excluded.) An immediate operation was performed in the emergency room.
How should his algorithms be modified?

Total daily insulin requirement will probably increase by 50 to 100%. Therefore, the algorithms for both basal and prandial insulin substitution can be raised by at least 50%.

It would also be permissible to simply correct elevated blood sugar values during the first day or so (primary adjustment), and then decide on appropriate algorithm modifications on the second or third day (secondary adjustment).

As far as the patient is capable of rational action, he might undertake the following steps:

1. At least a rough estimation of previous average daily insulin requirement (from self-monitoring records);
2. Rough calculation of current daily insulin requirement (including amounts needed for corrections);
3. Setting up the quotient:

$$\frac{\text{Current daily insulin requirement}}{\text{Previous daily insulin requirement}}$$

4. Multiplying the previous (successful) basal and prandial algorithms by this quotient to obtain the new dosage guidelines.

days, drastic reduction of caloric intake (e.g., to below 600–700 kcal per day) results in a reduction of basal insulin requirement (apparently due to reduced hepatic glucose production and decreased glycogen stores) to about 40–50% of the original requirement. The morning increase in basal requirements also disappears!

Blood sugar values during the day are not suitable for evaluating the accuracy of the basal rate. Interference arises from numerous factors, including regular insulin doses, carbohydrate intake and physical activity. Nighttime hypoglycemia is also not a good criterion, since it is more often due to an evening dose of regular insulin than to an excessive basal rate.

Basal insulin dosage can be best evaluated on the basis of the following criteria (see Sect. 5.1):

1. **Stability of blood glucose during short-term fasting (overnight or between meals);**
2. **Fasting blood glucose (target: 90–140 mg/dl);**
3. **Ratio of delayed to regular insulin over 24 h (35–50%).**

8.2.2 Modifying the Algorithms for Prandial Insulin

The following situations indicate that the algorithms for dosing prandial insulin are too low; i.e., the amount of insulin injected for one carbohydrate unit should be increased (by 20% as a first step):

- Repeatedly elevated late post-prandial blood glucose values (at least 3 hours – or even later – after the injection of regular insulin. Before modifying the algorithm, however, it should be determined whether blood glucose was already elevated when food was consumed. If so, glucose transport would be extremely slow and blood glucose might remain elevated for 4–6 hours, even if the patient had included a "correction" for the hyperglycemia in his preprandial injection of regular insulin. Hyperglycemia due to inappropriate insulin absorption kinetics (e.g., more rapid absorption of carbohydrates than of insulin, inadequate interval between injecting and eating) must also be excluded.
- Relatively low proportion of regular insulin to total daily dose.

The following situations indicate that the prandial algorithms are too high, i.e., the amount of insulin injected for one carbohydrate unit:

- Repeated hypoglycemic episodes. Here it must be taken into account that with a relative overdose of prandial insulin, hypoglycemia may not occur until a number of hours after the injection, especially if the meal was a large one. Inappropriate corrections with regular insulin and incorrect estimates of nutrient quantity, etc., also need to be excluded.
- A further indication that prandial insulin dosage is too high is a consistently large proportion of regular insulin (i.e., over 70%) in the total daily dose.

8.2.3 Modifying the Algorithms for Correcting Blood Glucose Excursions

The algorithms for correction describe the predictability of blood glucose dynamics after carbohydrate intake or administration of regular insulin. They are valid only under the condition that basal insulin dosage is correct. The difficulties in achieving basal conditions were discussed in Sect. 4.6 about determining the kidney threshold. Basal conditions can really only be said to exist when blood glucose, insulin level and insulin sensitivity are all stable, there is no renal loss of glucose and no relevant carbohydrate absorption from the intestinal tract, and hepatic glucose production remains constant. It is practically impossible to achieve these conditions simultaneously in a type I diabetic patient, but for practical purposes they can be approximated well enough for the patient to arrive at useful algorithms:

- 1 unit (U) of regular insulin lowers my blood glucose (BG) by ... mg/dl = Change in BG (delta BG) produced by 1 U of regular insulin
- 1 carbohydrate unit (12 g) raises my blood glucose by ... mg/dl = Change in BG (delta BG) produced by one carbohydrate unit.

Change in BG per unit of regular insulin:
For a patient with a body weight of approx. 60 kg and a daily insulin requirement of 40–60 units, one unit of regular insulin lowers blood sugar by approx. 40 mg/dl. The absolute value of delta BG would be greater for a patient who weighed less (one unit would produce a greater change) and smaller for someone who weighed more.

The value of **delta BG per unit of regular insulin** in the algorithm **should be increased** under the following conditions:

- Lowered total daily insulin requirement (e.g., increased physical activity, after childbirth, etc.);
- As a precaution at the beginning of FIT, since patients do not yet have a good grasp of insulin action at this point and may make incorrect dosage decisions;
- If the patient has a history of severe hypoglycemia (H3), is otherwise at risk of hypoglycemia, or is currently in a situation with a high risk of hypoglycemia (see Chap. 6, "Hypoglycemia");
- At very high blood glucose levels, where large amounts of glucose are being lost in the urine. (Since no insulin is required for the transport of glucose lost in the urine, there is danger of overdosing regular insulin when making corrections at severe hyperglycemic levels. However, a longer period of hyperglycemia will induce an insuline resistance).
- If the patient has a very low kidney threshold, since here again, no insulin is required for the glucose lost in the urine.

Conversely, the value of delta BG per unit of regular insulin **should be decreased** in the algorithm if the following situations apply:

- If total daily insulin requirement is high or on the increase;
- For i.v. insulin administration (in exceptional situations).

Change in BG per carbohydrate unit:
The change in BG produced by one unit of carbohydrates is mainly determined by current insulin level and the absorption kinetics of the particular carbohydrate. Its value should be decreased *in the algorithm if the following situations apply:*

- High rate of basal insulin ("eating to keep up with the basal rate" is necessary);
- Excellent residual function of beta cells;
- Large distribution volume (high body weight);
- Slowly absorbed carbohydrates.

Conversely, **the value of delta BG per carbohydrate unit should be increased** in the following situations:

- Low rate of basal insulin (underdosed, with tendency toward ketonuria);

- Small volume of distribution (low body weight)
- For psychological - not metabolic - reasons, when a patient tends to eat without injecting insulin.

8.2.4 Modifying the Target Values for Current Blood Glucose and Target Range for Mean Blood Glucose

In practice, it is important to note the difference between the target values for correction of hyperglycemia (fasting, postprandial, before going to bed) and the target range for mean blood glucose (MBG). These values play a very important role in the feedback loop of "control of glycemia by patients." The reasons for changing the blood glucose target value for corrections are seldom metabolic in nature; changes are most often necessary for patients with a history of severe hypoglycemia. The usual target value for corrections is 100 mg/dl for fasting and preprandial blood glucose and up to 180 mg/dl for postprandial measurements.

These target values should be raised (e.g., to 110-130 mg/dl for fasting and preprandial values and up to 200 mg/dl for postprandial measurements) under the following conditions:

- In situations that increase (temporarily) the risk of hypoglycemia;
- For patients whose characteristics increase the risk of hypoglycemia. The greater the number of high-risk characteristics a patient has, (see Chap. 6, "Hypoglycemia"), the higher his target range should be set.

There is rarely a reason to lower the blood glucose target values for constant corrections to below 100 mg/dl for fasting and preprandial measurements or to below 160 mg/dl for postprandial measurements. Lower targets can be set only when the patient has **no history of severe hypoglycemia**. The target points for correction of hyperglycemia are lowered during pregnancy. During the last 3 months of pregnancy, fasting and preprandial targets should be particularly low, at about 85 mg. Although blood glucose values between 65 and 85 mg/dl would otherwise be corrected to avoid hypoglycemia, they are not corrected during the last 3 months of pregnancy if there are no symptoms. During this period the postprandial target for the correction of hyperglycemia is set at 120 mg/dl (see also Chap. 10 on pregnancy). It may be advantageous for patients with an extremely low kidney threshold (e.g., around 110 mg/dl) to use 90 mg/dl as a target for fasting and preprandial blood glucose, since otherwise there would be too great a loss of urinary glucose. Very occasionally, a lower target might be useful for psychological reasons, especially for patients who without any rational reason seem to prefer hyperglycemia (and who tend to underdose insulin), such as is sometimes the case with adolescents.

It is necessary to differentiate between the target values for the correction of hyperglycemia - which the patient compares with the actual value at each blood glucose determination - and the target range for mean blood glucose. The mean blood glucose of the day is an important basis for the secondary adjustment of the insulin dosage. Approximately one third of the values used to calculate the mean blood glucose of the day (MBG) should be postprandial determinations. Patients with normal hypoglycemia awareness record possible hypoglycemic episodes as 40 mg/dl for the purpose of calculation, even when no actual blood glucose determination was carried out. The MBG achieved by patients is approximately 20-50 mg/dl higher than the target value they use for fasting and preprandial correction of hyperglycemia. Based on previous studies we can assume that the daily MBG calculated from self-monitored values is approximately 10-20 mg/dl lower than actual blood glucose levels.

For the majority of patients with type I diabetes the ideal target range for the daily MBG is from 110 (120) to approximately 160 (170) mg/dl (DCCT Research Group 1991, 1993), a compromise aimed at lowering the risk of hypoglycemia as much as possible, while limiting the risk of microvascular damage. If the MBG exceeds or fails to reach this target range over *several consecutive* days, then the relevant algorithms should be adjusted accordingly.

Patients who have been hyperglycemic may have a particularly acute awareness of hypoglycemia and thus may not be willing to accept a low target range for their MBG. In such cases it is advisable to suggest a higher than usual target range at first. Even for patients with advanced microvascular complications (for example, proliferative retinopathy requiring laser coagulation), it is better to start with a target MBG range of 140-180 mg/dl, for example, which can then be gradually lowered.

It is definitely necessary to lower the MBG target range during pregnancy. If possible (i.e., if the patient has no history of hypoglycemia), it would be acceptable to set the MBG target range to under 100 mg/dl during organogenesis (week 5 until approximately week 9 after the last menstruation; for patients with a history of severe hypoglycemia, a range under 120 mg/dl would be acceptable. However, the target range should be further lowered during the third trimester, when the mother's level of metabolic control determines the extent of neonatal complications. After approximately the 28th week of pregnancy at the latest, the MBG should be lowered to under 90 mg/dl, or if possible, even under 85 mg/dl (Howorka et al. 1996).

The period of partial remission after the initial manifestation of diabetes is another situation in which it may be desirable to set a very low target range for the MBG. Tight control of glycemia during this period may possibly aid in preserving residual beta cell function, and the risk of serious hypoglycemia is still low.

8.2.5 Interdependence of Algorithms

The values of the algorithms used for FIT are dependent upon each other. Assuming that the total daily insulin requirement remains relatively constant, if the basal rate (or its delayed-acting component) is lowered, then the values of the algorithms for prandial insulin (or for the regular insulin component of the basal rate) will be greater (more insulin will be needed per carbohydrate unit), and the drop in blood glucose per unit of insulin in the algorithm for correction will be correspondingly less.

Conversely, if the basal rate is set too high (allowing part of the prandial insulin requirement to be covered by the delayed-acting insulin), the values of the prandial algorithms must be lowered, and the probability of a "spontaneous" drop in blood sugar is increased. The value of delta BG (drop in blood glucose per unit of insulin) in the algorithm for correction with regular insulin would need to be greater. (In the extreme case, the patient would also have to "eat to keep up with the basal rate"; carbohydrate consumption would hardly raise blood sugar, even if no prandial insulin were injected. See Sect. 5.1, "Basal Substitution.")

9 Physical Activity

Physical activity usually reduces insulin requirement. The degree of reduction is dependent on current level of insulinemia, duration and intensity of physical activity.

A number of attempts have already been made to set up rules for insulin-treated diabetic patients to use in adjusting their insulin dose, carbohydrate intake, and level of physical activity in order to maintain good metabolic control (Schiffrin et al. 1985; Sonnenberg et al. 1984). These rules are not directly applicable to the practice of FIT, however. One reason is that they are generally based on physical activity that takes place soon after eating (when the level of prandial insulin is still relatively high). They are also based on therapy regimes which assume a relatively uniform diet and conventional insulin dosage.

Under normal living conditions, the biggest difficulties for the patient arise from the fact that it is rarely possible to know ahead of time exactly how intense physical activity will be and how long it will last. The phenomenon of "planned exercise" is apparently rare (Schiffrin 1985). The ordinary spurts of physical activity in daily life are just as unplanned for the diabetic patient as they are for anyone else. For the type I diabetic patient this means, however, that it is very difficult, if not impossible, to plan ahead sufficiently to make the necessary changes in his insulin dosage.

The following recommendations for accommodating carbohydrate intake and insulin dosage to physical activity attempt to take this common problem of **unplanned** activity into account. They are based mainly on clinical experience rather than controlled experimental studies, although available scientific evidence has, of course, been considered.

Basically, we need to differentiate between sporadic (unplanned) spurts of physical activity and longer periods lasting over several days.

9.1 Short, Sporadic Periods of Physical Activity

For sporadic increases in activity, the current level of insulinemia (i.e., time interval since the last injection of regular insulin) needs to be taken into account.

9.1.1 Physical Activity not Preceded by a Recent Injection of Regular Insulin

If the current level of insulin in the blood results from the basal rate alone, i.e., when the period of physical activity begins four or five hours after eating – or more exactly, after the prandial insulin injection – then the recommendation is to consume extra, easily-absorbable carbohydrates in the amount of **one carbohydrate unit (12 g) for each 45–60 minutes of moderate physical activity** (approx. 40–50% of the VO_2 max.).

If the patient uses an insulin infusion pump, he should also consume a small amount of carbohydrates (approx. one carbohydrate unit) when physical activity takes place long after the last preprandial bolus. Interrupting the continuous insulin infusion is also helpful.

9.1.2 Physical Activity after Regular Insulin

After an injection of regular insulin, or an insulin bolus from an infusion pump, levels of insulin in the blood are fairly high. This results in an even stronger inhibition of hepatic glucose production than would be produced by the basal rate alone. Thus, approx. one "insulin-free" carbohydrate unit would be necessary for each 20–30 minutes of moderate physical activity. It must be emphasized that only truly "extra" carbohydrates (for which no prandial insulin is administered) are meant here. It is immaterial whether the patient consumes an extra meal without prandial insulin or simply eats his usual amount just before the beginning of the activity and reduces his insulin dose accordingly.

With an insulin infusion pump, prompt interruption of insulin flow is possible. Here the patient should still eat one or two carbohydrate units at the beginning of the activity period and interrupt the insulin infusion as well.

9.1.3 Further Influences

Other factors also need to be considered during physical activity in type I diabetes. The *intensity* of the exercise is important. Physical activity that begins abruptly and continues at high intensity (tennis, running etc.) may result in a paradoxical increase in blood glucose. This effect may also be particularly intensified by the presence of even slight hypoinsulinemia, which is normally negligible, occurring without ketonuria and recognizable simply by slightly increased blood glucose values (130 mg/dl). On the other hand, physical activity may also have a lasting "delayed effect" on insulin requirements; even many hours after physical exercise has ended, insulin sensitivity may be improved and insulin requirement decreased. Therefore, insulin dosage should be kept low just after exercise (and also for a number of hours afterwards). This effect is more pronounced with relatively high basal insulinization and larger muscle mass.

9.2 Prolonged Periods of Physical Activity

Prolonged periods of physical exercise can normally be planned. The total basal and prandial insulin dosage should be reduced beforehand to about 40–60% of the usual requirement (secondary adjustment = correction of algorithms). When ultralente (or even lente) insulins are used for basal substitution, however, their long half-life results in a delay of at least one day (12 hours or more) before the effects of a reduction in dosage are felt. This could be a distinct disadvantage in the secondary adjustment of insulin dosage to compensate for physical activity, since it makes the system relatively sluggish. Fortunately, however, primary adjustments can be made to compensate for physical activity, so that in practice this disadvantage is hardly relevant.

On the first day of a period of strenuous physical exercise – much more intensive than usual – **the rules concerning carbohydrate intake during sporadic activity can be applied.** In concrete terms, this means that on the first day of such a period, the patient would probably inject very little regular insulin and would consume a relatively large amount of carbohydrates. He would consume 1–2 carbohydrate units per hour of exercise, the exact amount depending on his current insulin level (i.e., depending on when and how much insulin was injected) and the intensity of the activity). If, for example, he spends a day cross-country skiing (6–7 hours of relatively strenuous activity), he would consume about 10 or more units of "insulin-free" carbohydrates, distributed over the day. If he did not want to eat more than this amount, he would inject no regular insulin at all; his insulin requirements for the day would covered by the basal rate. He would, of course, monitor his blood sugar before, after, and even during the period of activity and make any necessary corrections.

On the second and following days, he would use the rules for secondary adaptation of insulin dosage to make the proper modifications in all of his algorithms (basal, prandial, and algorit hms for correction; see Chap. 8, "Rules for algorithm modification"). He would first determine his current insulin requirement, compare it to his daily insulin consumption before the period of physical activity began and adjust the algorithms proportionally to the new conditions of insulin sensitivity. That is, they would be reduced in proportion to the reduction of total daily dose, or in concrete terms, according to the following ratio:

$$\frac{\text{current daily insulin dose (IU)}}{\text{mean previous daily insulin dose (IU)}}$$

He would then use the criteria described in Chap. 8 ("Rules for Algorithm Modification") to test the validity of the adjustments.

Since the effects of physical exercise on actual insulin requirement cannot really be predicted with accuracy, the importan ce of frequent blood glucose monitoring must be emphasized (before, after, and even during the activity). The patients should also be well-informed about the prolonged effects of physical activity which result in danger of hypoglycemia during the night following the exercise.

If a patient has an absolute insulin deficiency (hyperglycemia, ketosis), physical activity will lead to a worsening of the metabolic situation (Berger et al. 1977). If the exercise is initially very strenuous, this will also aggravate hyperglycemia. The insulin deficiency should therefore be eliminated before undertaking physical activity.

10 Pregnancy in Type I (Insulin-Dependent) Diabetes

10.1 Patient Education Concerning Diabetes and Pregnancy

Information on the following points is obligatory:

- **Risks for the Child**

Perinatal mortality in children of diabetic mothers is a function of maternal glycemia during pregnancy (Jovanovic and Peterson 1980). Maternal hyperglycemia during the phase of organ development (first trimester) leads to an increase in the risk of malformation. During the further course of pregnancy, especially during the third trimester, it causes reactive fetal hyperinsulinemia, which leads to macrosomia and pronounced hypoglycemia in the newborn. Optimal metabolic control from the beginning of the pregnancy can almost completely eliminate the excessive perinatal mortality of children of diabetic mothers (Fuhrmann et al. 1983, Miller et al. 1983).

- **Probability of Diabetes in Children of Diabetic Mothers**

Contrary to previous beliefs, the probability that a child of a type I diabetic mother will also develop diabetes is very low, approx. 1–3% (Warram et al. 1984).

- **Risk for the Diabetic Mother**

Any existing late complications of diabetes increase the risk to both mother and child. Angiopathy multiplies the risk of late gestosis (preeclampsia). Care should therefore be especially intensive if any of the following conditions are present:

- long duration of diabetes (and/or early manifestation of diabetes in the mother);
- retinopathy;

- nephropathy (increased microproteinuria, hypertension, pyelonephritis).

10.2 Consequences for Treatment

Any pregnancy in a type I (insulin-dependent) diabetic patient is a high-risk pregnancy. Only optimal metabolic control during the entire pregnancy can reduce the risk to the child. From a public health standpoint, all diabetic women of child-bearing age should be given the opportunity to take part in a comprehensive diabetes education program, plus sufficient information on birth control (low-dose ovulation inhibitors, barrier methods, etc.) and on the necessity for planning of pregnancy.

In order to reduce the potential risk to a minimum and to achieve an optimal course of pregnancy, complete cooperation between a diabetologist, an obstetrician and an ophthalmologist is necessary. This is generally available only in a specialized treatment center. Comprehensive neonatal care must also be available.

10.3 Interdisciplinary Care for Pregnant Diabetic Women

The goals of interdisciplinary care are to achieve normoglycemia both before conception and during the entire course of the pregnancy, including during childbirth, to minimize hospital stays, and as far as possible to enable a normal, full-term, vaginal birth. The ultimate goal is naturally a healthy child.

10.3.1 Diabetological Care: FIT

There is probably no better indication for FIT than pregnancy in a diabetic woman. Except when complications are present, patients preconceptionally trained in FIT rarely need to be hospitalized during pregnancy (see Sect. 16.4, "Experience with FIT in special situations"). Pregnancy under FIT simply leads to the following (relatively slight) changes in therapeutic goals and measures:

- **Self-Monitoring**

The time and effort expended for self-monitoring should be doubled during pregnancy (from approx. 10 minutes per day, normally, to approx. 20 minutes per day in pregnancy). The number of blood sugar measurements should not be less than 6 per day. Contrary to usual practice under FIT, the emphasis should be on postprandial values (1–2 hours after eating). The urine should also be tested for acetone much more frequently than usual – daily, if there is vomiting or if food intake is restricted in order to prevent excessive weight gain.

- **Blood Glucose Target Points for Constant Corrections and Target Range for MBG**

If the patient has no history of severe hypoglycemia, the blood glucose target values should be lowered to 90 mg/dl for preprandial and 120 (140) mg/dl for postprandial values. Although a weekly mean blood glucose (MBG) of 140–150 mg/dl can be acceptable in a non-pregnant diabetic woman, during pregnancy MBG should be under 100 mg/dl (or under 120 mg/dl for patients at risk for hypoglycemia). During the last trimester of pregnancy, the mother's glycemic control determines the extent of any potential neonatal complications specific to diabetes (macrosomia, hypoglycemia etc.). From week 28 onwards, the daily mean blood glucose should be lowered to under 90 or even approximately 85 mg/dl. The probability of severe hypoglycemia is relatively low because of the physiological insulin resistance that exists during this period. To achieve a mean blood glucose under 90 mg/dl, the patient should use the following target points for correcting hyperglycemia: 85 mg/dl for fasting and preprandial hyperglycemia and up to 120 mg/dl for correcting postprandial hyperglycemia (Howorka et al. 1996). Furthermore, during pregnancy, blood sugar values just above the hypoglycemic range (70–90 mg/dl) are not corrected with additional carbohydrate intake as they otherwise would be under FIT. The calculation of a daily and weekly MBG is essential (See Sect. 5.3.1, "Record Keeping, Analysis and Evaluation of the Daily Net Result"). Glycosylated hemoglobin should also be maintained in the lower normal range.

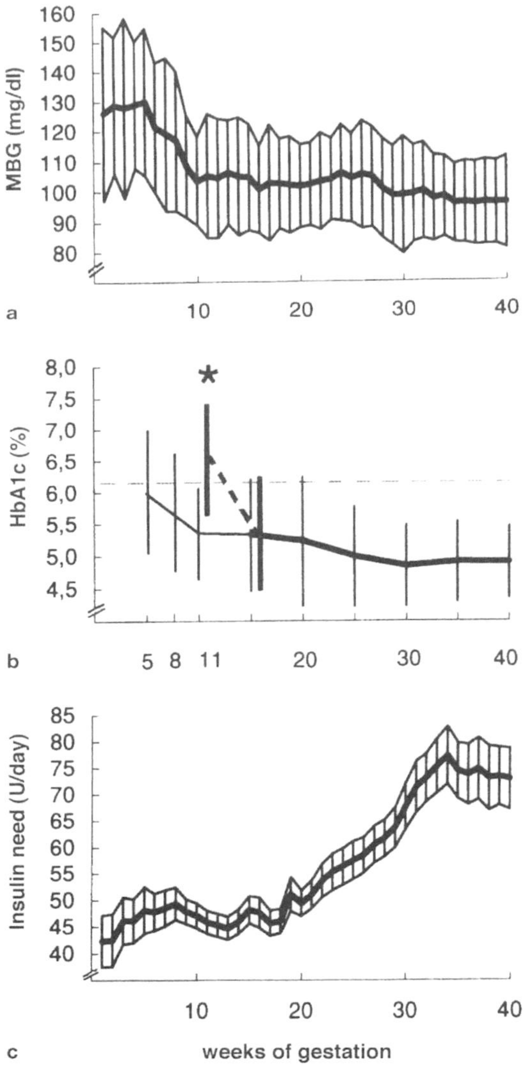

Fig. 10.1.a (top): Weekly mean blood glucose (mean ± SD) during pregnancy for 58 female patients under functional insulin treatment. The lowering of MBG in the 5th–6th week can be attributed to the motivating effect of a positive pregnancy test
b Course of HbA_{1c} values (mean ± SD, normal range up to 6.1%) in pregnant diabetic women. Women who had FIT-training before conception **(thin lines)** had significantly lower HbA_{1c} values at week 11–12 than women who began functional insulin treatment at week 11 ± 3 **(dotted line)**; * $p < 0.009$
c The course of insulin requirements (mean ± SEM) during pregnancy in insulin-dependent functionally treated diabetic women (Howorka et al. 1996)

- **Frequency of Hypoglycemia**

Contrary to earlier fears, there is no evidence that maternal hypoglycemia harms the fetus. Since severe hypoglycemia (grades H2, H3) can be a danger to the mother, however – just as for any non-pregnant diabetic patient – it should be avoided.

- **Insulin Administration**

As for non-pregnant diabetic patients, multiple insulin injections and CSII can achieve comparable levels of glycemic control during pregnancy (Coustan et al., 1986). Due to their high motivation, however, pregnant patients are especially easy to persuade to use an infusion device.

- **Special Aspects of Motivation**

Assuming opportunities for adequate patient education, the care of pregnant diabetic patients is one of the easiest and most pleasant tasks a diabetologist can have. In contrast to non-pregnant diabetic patients, there is hardly ever a problem in motivating the patient to strive for good metabolic control. The greatest advantage of FIT for the non-diabetic patient is the flexibility of lifestyle that it offers, but for the pregnant diabetic woman, the well-being of the child is the most important motivating factor. Therefore, even very intensive and/or difficult measures such as frequent self-monitoring, prolonging the interval between eating and injecting, eating relatively regular meals, daily analysis of food intake and insulin administration, etc., are taken gladly into account by patients who have undergone training in FIT.

- **General Internal Supervision**

Due to the improvements in therapy, pregnancy is now possible in spite of even advanced late complications. Proper care of a pregnant diabetic woman with a high risk of preeclampsia due to late complications includes regular and frequent monitoring of blood pressure, microalbuminuria and kidney function. Possibilities for therapy of hypertension include methyldopa, hydralazine, atenolol, and metoprolol. Patients with hypertension should complete an antihypertensive patient education program before attempting to become pregnant. Particular attention should be paid to infections of the urinary tract. Weight gain should be carefully monitored. Checks should also be made for the presence of edema of the legs at each visit.

Patients who have been trained in FIT before conception need no prophylactic hospitalization as long as outpatient visits are frequent. Ideally, weekly, or at least biweekly visits should be made to a specialized outpatient clinic. Within the framework of interdisciplinary care, the diabetologist takes over the task of coordinating the obstetrical, ophthalmological and other necessary examinations and measures, besides being responsible for patient education and general medical care.

- **Birth Preparation Course for Pregnant Diabetic Women and Their Partners**

The FIT group training uses preconceptional counseling and motivational techniques to lower the rate of malf ormation. To prepare the women and their partners for the last 3 months of pregnancy, as well as for delivery, breast-feeding and motherhood with diabetes, we have established a special, 1-day group course along with a parent/child center. This procedure has enabled us to achieve results for diabetic pregnancies comparable to those in a healthy population (Howorka et al. 1995). In addition to intensive treatment, our explicit aim was to offer our patients the greatest possible opportunity for conscious self-determination, before, during and after the birth, while taking the existing risk and the undeniable necessity of intensive orthodox medical supervision into account.

The main points covered in this program include glycemic control in normal pregnancy, blood glucose targets in diabetic pregnancy, especially during the period after the 24th week of pregnancy, when the risk of hypoglycemia decreases, the connection between daily insulin requirements and the function of the placenta, proteinuria and hypertension, the pathophysiology of maternal hypoglycemia/fetal hyperinsulinemia, prevention of excessive increases in maternal weight, possibilities and indications for induction of birth, secondary insulin dosage adaptation before and after birth, heredity and diabetes under particular consideration of breast feeding versus early exposure to cow's milk. Wherever possible, potential functions of the partner during each phase of pregnancy are discussed in detail; for example, how to motivate the expectant mother, helping her to monitor and record blood glucose, how to prevent and treat hypoglycemia, the possibilities for and meaning of his concrete help during each phase of childbirth, as well as the statistical probability of postnatal depression and ways of preventing or ameliorating it. The patients learn that after the start of contractions, the FIT algorithms are reduced to one third of their previous values, and their partners are motivated to help them monitor blood glucose at least every 2 h during the opening phase.

10.3.2 Obstetrical Care

Obstetrical care should include approximately 11–12 visits up to the due date. Besides external and internal examinations, ultrasound biometry should be used to follow parameters of fetal growth. Skull and abdomen diameter, as well as femur length should be measured and documented on corresponding growth curves. The sonographic examination should be complemented by examinations of placental position and morphology, estimation of amount of amniotic fluid, and thorough examination of fetal organ systems as an extended screening for malformation (wk 20–23). A cardiotocogram and tests of placental function, e.g., HPL (human placental lactogen), estriol, oxytocin stress test, are important during the third trimester. Nonstress tests (NST) and a "biophysical profile" have now become routine.

Just as for nondiabetic women, participation in a course on preparation for childhood (if possible, with the partner) should be strongly recommended.

10.3.3 Ophthalmological Care

Since the status of retinopathy is a factor in deciding the method of delivery, especially in patients with advanced late complications, ophthalmological care takes on great importance, particularly the early focal or panretinal coagulation of neovascularization. At least three ophthalmological examinations should be made during the course of pregnancy.

10.3.4 Neonatal Care

Due to the risk of malformation, macrosomia and hypoglycemia in a diabetic pregnancy, specialized neonatological care may be necessary. Experience shows, however, that hardly any relevant complications – particularly not hypoglycemia – occur in children of mothers who have achieved near-normal glycemic levels throughout pregnancy.

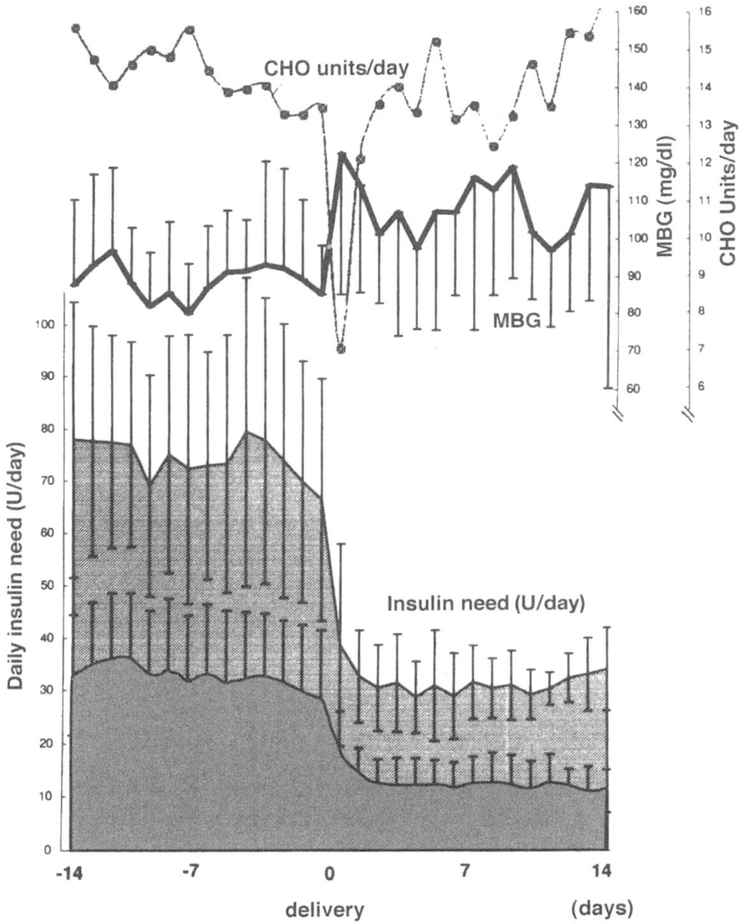

Fig. 10.2. Carbohydrate intake, mean blood glucose (MBG), and insulin requirements before, during, and after childbirth in type I diabetic women under functional insulin treatment (mean ± SD). **Dark shading**, delayed-acting insulin; **light shading**, regular insulin. These data are from the subgroup of patients with vaginal delivery, **n** = 18 (Howorka et al. 1996)

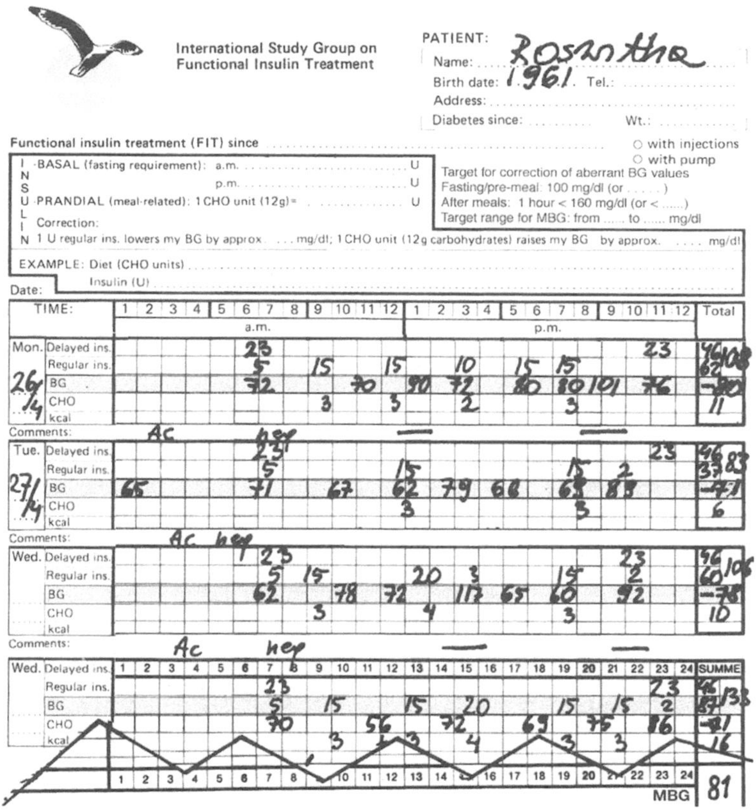

Fig. 10.3. A pregnant diabetic patient has had functional insulin treatment during the last trimester of pregnancy.
Which steps has she undertaken to achieve optimal glycemic control? Would these also be applicable outside of pregnancy?
Which dosage guidelines would you suggest during childbirth?

Answer: Basal: ....

Prandial: ....

Correction of hyperglycemia: ....

Reason?

The patient has taken the following steps:

- Monitors her blood glucose very frequently, including postprandial determinations
- Has lowered her target for correction of hyperglycemia, fasting as well as postprandial
- Accepts blood glucose values between 70 and 85 mg/dl without correction
- Has lowered her MBG target range to under 90 mg/dl
- Tests her urine regularly for acetone (She has had to reduce her calorie intake be cause she has already gained 15 kg in weight.)
- Records any periods where her preprandial blood glucose is above her target range in her logbook, which keeps her on her toes.

Such strict procedures are only recommended during pregnancy, when insulin resistance is present. These recommendations are not applicable to normal conditions, when insulin resistance is not present!

This patient is highly motivated because she has previously gone through two complicated pregnancies while under conventional therapy. Her first child had macrosomia, and her second also had macrosomia and was stillborn.

During delivery she reduces her insulin dosage as follows:
With the start of contractions, there is likely to be a decrease in insulin requirement. She therefore reduces the values in her prandial and basal algorithms to one third of their previous values.

Suggestion for new algorithms (during delivery and immediately afterwards)

Basal:	mornings 7 IU ultralente insulin + 2 IU regular insulin late evenings 7 IU NPH insulin
Prandial:	1.5 IU regular insulin per carbohydrate unit
Correction:	Delta – BG for every 1 IU = –40 mg/dl

In order to avoid hypoglycemia, the target value for correction of hyperglycemia should be increased to 100 mg/dl during delivery and further increased to approximately 120 mg/dl afterwards.

Since her insulin requirements will change again in the days or weeks following delivery, she will then need to carry out another secondary adjustment, i.e., she will need to change her algorithms again to adjust to the new situation.

Routine hospitalization of the newborn on a neonatological ward just because the mother has diabetes is therefore no longer justified. Repeated blood glucose measurements during the first 24 hours after birth must be possible, however. It should also be pointed out that, after months of strenuous cooperation during an entire pregnancy, diabetic mothers deserve to spend the time immediately after childbirth with their infants. Brestfeeding should be supported.

10.4 Special Aspects of Secondary Adjustment of Insulin Dosage During Pregnancy and Childbirth

For unexplained reasons, insulin requirement usually falls slightly during the first trimester of pregnancy and then rises again during the 12th to 14th week, due to the increased counter-effects of placental hormones (progesterone, HPL, estriol). Insulin requirement reaches a maximum (from 50% to 300% higher than before conception) toward the end of pregnancy. After childbirth it falls drastically to only 30–50% of the values at the end of pregnancy. It then rises again (usually after a few weeks) to preconceptional levels. Patients naturally need to be informed of the necessity for secondary adjustment of algorithms during pregnancy. They also need to be informed that a sudden drop in insulin requirement during pregnancy could be an indication of placental insufficiency or intrauterine fetal death. However, the marked drop in insulin requirement that is usually seen in about 50% of patients during the last weeks (or days) of pregnancy, indicates a physiological loss of placental function.

Insulin substitution during childbirth is relatively simple for FIT-trained patients. At the beginning of contractions, the algorithms for basal and prandial insulin are reduced to about 30% (up to 50%) of the previous value, to accommodate the expected drop in insulin requirement. If contractions start after the injection of the usual dose of delayed-acting insulin, basal insulinization will be too high, so additional glucose should be administered (approx. 30g, maximum of 40g), either intravenously or orally. Normoglycemia during the birth is easily obtainable with blood glucose tests every one to two hours. If secondary adjustment of algorithms can be made in time, no glucose infusion is necessary. As a precaution, however, preparations for intravenous infusion should be made.

11 Functional Insulin Treatment for Type II Diabetes

11.1 Characteristics of Treatment of Type II Diabetes

Originally (at the beginning of the 1980s), functional insulin treatment was basically conceived of as substitution of insulin deficiency to achieve near-normal glycemia in type I diabetic patients. Many type II diabetic patients, however, soon showed an interest in this new form of therapy. Its two main advantages, the flexibility of food intake and the potential for immediate correction of hyperglycemia, are also relevant to type II diabetic patients who are treated with insulin, even though they are not insulin-dependent.

Over the years, therefore, we have often integrated type II diabetic patients who wish to have functional insulin treatment into our courses along with type I diabetic patients. In our experience, these patients generally differ from type I diabetic patients in the following ways:

1. Due to insulin resistance and/or residual insulin secretion, their diabetes tends to be less brittle, i.e., their blood glucose does not fluctuate as widely as that of type I diabetic patients.
2. The risk of severe hypoglycemia is less. Their otherwise undesirable insulin resistance exercises a certain protective function here.
3. Since type II diabetic patients usually present at an older age than type I patients (usually in their 60s or 70s, although many patients do manifest in their 30s, 40s or 50s), they tend to learn more slowly than type I patients, who generally enter our program in their younger age.

The fact that good glycemic control is easier to achieve for type II diabetics tends to compensate for their somewhat slower rate of learning, so that at least if certain guidelines are followed, type I and II diabetics can be integrated in the same group with no difficulty.

11.2 Covering Basal Insulin Requirements in Insulin-Treated Type II Diabetic Patients

Type II diabetics commonly are able to produce relatively large amounts of insulin, but due to insulin resistance, their endogenous insulin is not sufficient to achieve optimal postprandial glycemic control, after carbohydrate intake. The amount of endogenous insulin secretion can be determined by measuring insulin levels in patients who have not yet been treated with insulin, or by measuring basal C-peptide in patients already on insulin. Depending on the severity of the diabetes and the level of fasting blood glucose values, functional insulin treatment can be undertaken varying degrees of coverage of basal insulin requirement.

- **No Substitute for the Basal Requirement**

When the basal insulin requirement is low, it may be possible to optimize glycemic control simply by administering regular insulin to cover prandial needs and for correction of spontaneous hyperglycemia. This form of treatment is easy to introduce under outpatient conditions, since patients need only learn the prandial rule, "How many units of insulin per carbohydrate unit," and the rule for correction of hyperglycemia, "1 unit of regular insulin lowers my blood glucose by..." If fasting hyperglycemia should occur under this form of therapy (fasting blood glucose values over approximately 150 mg/dl), additional therapeutic measures are necessary, whether with oral antidiabetic agents or delayed-acting insulin.

- **Biguanides to Help Cover the Basal Requirement**

Biguanides work mainly by inhibiting hepatic glucose production. This form of therapy has found increasing acceptance, especially with *overweight* diabetic patients. Biguanides do not induce hypoglycemia. They also have an additional (desirable) appetite-depressant effect. Biguanides can be used in combination with insulin and, if insulin resistance is present, also contribute to decreasing the insulin requirements. If good control of fasting hyperglycemia can be achieved with biguanides, regular insulin can be administered to cover prandial needs and correct hyperglycemia as usual under FIT.

A very rare, but nonetheless sometimes deadly complication of biguanide therapy is lactic acidosis, which may occur if kidney function is impaired. Biguanides should thus be used only when kidney function is normal (creatinine < 1.4 mg/dl).

• **Coverage of the Basal Insulin Requirement Using Sulfonylureas**
Another option for therapy of type II diabetes is the combination of a long-acting sulfonylurea (for example, glibenclamide) with regular insulin for meals. The use of sulfonylureas is not without risk, since if severe hypoglycemia does occur, the prognosis is considerably worse than that of hypoglycemia produced by insulin. Furthermore, the use of regular insulin to correct hyperglycemic values becomes problematical under sulfonylureas, since blood glucose may drop "spontaneously." The treatment for hypoglycemia under sulfonylurea therapy must be discussed in extensive detail with the patient. Intravenous glucose administration is necessary; glucogon is not suitable, particularly with long-acting sulfonylureas.

• **Delayed-acting Insulin for Coverage of the Basal Insulin Requirement in Type II Diabetes**
With clinically relevant insulin resistance and high insulin requirements, we generally recommend combining an ultralente insulin in the morning with an NPH or lente insulin in the late evening to cover basal needs. This combination allows control of fasting blood glucose with a relatively low dosage. As already explained in detail in the chapter on basal substitution, lente or NPH insulins should be administered late at night before going to bed, not before the evening meal.

Basal substitution can also be carried out by combining insulin with biguanides or sulfonylurea, particularly in the case of pronounced resistance to insulin. This enables the insulin dosage to be kept lower.

11.3 Special Aspects of the FIT Training Program for Type II Diabetic Patients

Younger type II diabetic patients generally are willing to monitor blood glucose several times daily, but often do not have the technical expertise to do so easily during their everyday routine. Therefore, the practical aspects of self-monitoring under everyday conditions are discussed during the basic diabetes education phase and the relevant skills practiced.

Since nutrition and the prevention of weight gain are of importance for the course of type II diabetes, these topics receive particular emphasis. Special attention is also paid to the various disorders besides impaired glucose tolerance which are associated with this metabolic syndrome (hyperinsulinemia, hypertension, and hypercholesterolemia).

Therefore, less is said about insulin deficiency per se and much more about the entire metabolic syndrome, its consequences, prognosis, and possibilities of treatment. It is evident that different subgroups of patients need specialized training, so in recent years we have developed the following supplementary outpatient education modules to be used in addition to the basic FIT training program:

(1) Training in the control of hypertension (3 evenings, see Chapter "Checklist for Continuing Care of FIT Patients - Late Complications")
(2) Training in the control of hyperlipidemia (2 evenings)
(3) Slimming course or weight loss support group (8 evenings at weekly intervals).

11.4 How Can Weight Loss Be Reached with Type II Diabetes During Functional Insulin Treatment

For patients with insulin resistance and abdominal obesity, weight loss is of decisive importance. FIT can be a significant help, since the patient who knows how to use it well is freed from having to eat to suit his insulin schedule.

A number of techniques appear to be useful in helping all types of diabetic patients to reduce their food intake and control their weight. Whatever method will be used, intensive physical exercise and self-monitoring of blood glucose and ketonuria are necessary. It is essential for patients to know how to adjust their insulin dosage and to take changes in requirements into account.

- **Special Low Calorie Days**

We have found it useful and relatively easy for patients to insert an occasional "vegetable and fruit day" into their schedules, a practice already recommended in the early 1900s by the diabetologist Carl von Noorden. On these days the patient eats only such foods as lettuce, raw or steamed vegetables, and fruit with as much liquid and roughage as possible (total caloric intake under approximately 400 kcal). Biguanides and sulfonylureas should be withdrawn and the insulin dosage halved. For patients on FIT, the basal insulin dose is halved and prandial insulin administration is maintained as usual. However, since caloric intake is much lower than usual, the amount of insulin needed to cover prandial needs is also much lower. Most patients are willing to accept a "vegetable and fruit day" once or twice a week.

- **Overall Reduction in Food Intake**
A conventional weight loss diet of under approximately 1200 kcal (fat and alcohol to be avoided) over a period of time also requires a corresponding reduction in insulin dosage. Delayed-acting insulin is usually reduced by 30% to 50%.

- **Fasting and Very Low Calorie Diets (VLCD)**
Modified forms of fasting have also proven to be successful in diabetic patients. The principle is the sole intake of large amounts of fluid in the form of "thinned" vegetable juices, vegetable broth, and teas. We have found a written "guide to fasting" and group support to be decisive in building up motivation.

Patients who work full time may find complete fasting to be too strenuous and may be more willing to stick to a "formula diet," of which there are many, in growing numbers, on the market. With this kind of "half-fasting," it is important that the patients themselves learn how to evaluate the nutritive content of the type they choose. They need to practice reading the labels and calculating the amount of carbohydrates and calories of their chosen "formula" in order to choose the right amount of insulin. Oral antidiabetic agents should also be omitted with this type of diet. If insulin is used to cover basal requirements, the dosage should be reduced to one third of usual, depending on the type of diabetes. In type II diabetes after a longer period of half-fasting, the basal insulin dose may be completely omitted.

All "radical" forms of dieting with diabetes require:

1. Information and motivation of the patient
2. Constant medical supervision, particularly with associated illnesses and pharmaco-therapies

3. Ongoing work with patients to help them improve both their lifestyle and eating habits. Education as to appropriate forms of *physical exercise* is also very important.

Group sessions seem to be the best and most efficient method of integrating these tasks and making them work for a large number of patients. (Our "slimming course" consists of 8 weekly meetings, then ongoing monthly get-togethers over a long period.)

With most patients the real goal is *not* a temporary loss of weight, which has a high probability of resulting in a "rebound" effect, but a lasting change in habits and lifestyle. In our experience, the most satisfactory results are achieved by combining behavior modification techniques (with emphasis on increasing physical activity (e.g., Wing et al. 1988; Kunze et al. 1991) with cognitive interventions such as educating patients about their condition and health risks, and about nutrition, balancing their diet, and reducing fat intake, and techniques of short-term cognitive therapy such as neurolinguistic programming (Besser-Siegmund 1992) or solution focus (de Shazer 1988). Patients in our "slimming course," where these levels of intervention are integrated, achieve a mean weight loss of 6 kg (range: 0–14 kg) in 4–5 months.

In summary, functional insulin treatment can be used successfully with type II diabetes and its flexibility offers a distinct advantage for the insulin-treated patients who need to lose weight. Either a special training course or training modules that supplement the usual FIT program (slimming-course, units on control of hyperlipidemia and hypertension) can be helpful with this group of patients.

12 Coping with Special Situations

Diverse rules of thumb have been suggested for patients under conventional insulin therapy for adapting their insulin regime to changing conditions in emergencies (Constam 1985) and in special situations such as managing insulin therapy when traveling across time zones, etc.

In our experience up to the present, diabetic patients under FIT are to a large extent immune to a variety of threatening occurrences because the FIT training enables them to cope with new situations.

The procedures we recommend can be summarized as follows. No really serious problems should occur as long as the patient is able (even if not optimally) to separately and independently:

(1) substitute basal insulin,
(2) substitute prandial insulin, and
(3) autonomously close the feedback loop by determining current glycemic levels and correcting them accordingly.

Both primary (correction of current off-target blood glucose values) and secondary (correction of algorithms) adjustments are decisive.

This procedure holds also for special situations such as hospital admissions (whether for surgery, childbirth, or any other reason). The experience of our patients has shown that trained diabetic patients know best themselves how to control their own blood sugar levels. As long as the patient is conscious and able to act rationally, he should be the one to make the decisions on insulin dosage. Even if he does not always make the ideal choice, **he will usually get better results than a new therapist, simply because, in contrast to even the best therapist, he is always available to himself;** he knows what his insulin dosage and algorithms have been, and he has enough practice to have acquired the corresponding skill in controlling his blood sugar. So whenever it is possible for th trained patient to maintain autonomy in "closing the open loop," he should be able to manage almost any potentially dangerous situation.

During the training program, a day or two after beginning functional insulin substitution, it is important to prepare patients for such situations by asking them to work out solutions to individually tailored hypothetical problems. For example, "Mark, imagine you are coming down with flu. You have fever and chills. What should you expect? What would you do, when and how? Think about it until tomorrow." ... "Elisabeth, let's assume that you have decided you want to get pregnant. Please tell us the day after tomorrow what you would do about your diabetes before and during pregnancy. What means of contraception might you have been using, and what would you do if you decided to stop? What sort of metabolic control would you be aiming at and how would you achieve it? What examinations would be important and when? What things would you have to consider before the due date?" ... "Mr. Mayer, you're a sportsman. Do you ski? Let's assume you're planning a skiing vacation in Austria. You'll be spending about 6 hours a day on the slopes. Please think about what you would do that would be different than usual. How would you do it?"

This procedure gives the individual patients a chance to participate actively in processing the theoretical material and helps make the complexities and interrelationships clear. Moreover, it helps motivate patients to select the sections of the teaching material that are relevant to themselves and their individual "special" situations. Further details are given in the patient handbook for FIT (K. Howorka, Kirchheim Publishers, Mainz 5th edition 1995). Interactions within the group are also enhanced, since it is much easier for participants to identify with and criticize each other than to analyze or even listen to recommendations made by a doctor (which are often not as practical anyway).

In order to make theoretical material (stress situations, short-term physical activity, late complications, etc.) meaningful to the patient, the essential skill needed by the doctor or trainer is to be able to pick situations that are individually relevant and that may actually happen to the individual participants (high school graduation, a tennis game, laser treatment, or whatever).

13 Frequent Patient-Related Problems

13.1 Grief-Work in Persons with Diabetes

Freud (1917) and Kübler-Ross (1969) differentiate three stages of working through grief after the loss of a loved one:

1. Denial of reality (Kübler-Ross also includes anger and negotiating);
2. Depression;
3. Acceptance and adjustment to the new reality.

Similar phases of grief-work also seem to be necessary after the loss of health, i.e., after the diagnosis of a chronic disease such as diabetes. From the standpoint of transactional analysis, these three phases might be thought of as corresponding to the three levels of personality: denial to the Child, depression to the Parent, and adjustment to the Adult. A healthy process of overcoming grief is indicated when the patient gives up the unrealistic expectation of "restitutio ad integrum" (complete restoration to health) in favor of the more realistic hope of "restitutio ad optimum" or restoration as far as is possible (Gfeller and Assal 1979).

One reason that FIT is so well accepted by patients is that it speeds up the process of rehabilitation. The prospect of achieving good metabolic control, which allows a high degree of biological integrity, ensures the cooperation of the Adult personality level. The wide flexibility of lifestyle and the opportunity for immediate response to current glycemic level ensures the cooperation of the Child level. Both the flexibility and the potentially greater independence from the physician, plus the greater social adaptability seem to offer additional psychosocial integrity that appeals to the Parent level.

The stages of grief-work are not necessarily consecutive. The patient may be adjusting to certain aspects of reality, while at the same time denying others. The adjustment to the reality of the disease and its phases (manifestation, therapy-related restrictions, late complications) should be seen as a dynamic, never-completed process. External influences may lead to a rapid regression from a state of acceptance to a predominance of denial or even self-destruction.

In considering errors made by patients, the mistakes that are due solely to ignorance need to be differentiated from those caused by incomplete adjustment to the realities of the disease. These may arise out of denial of reality or depression. It is not the Adult personality level that is responsible for such behavior, but rather either the archaic Child or the Parent. The diabetes counselor must be able to recognize and deal with such behavior in order to be effective.

13.2 Inadequate Information

Errors made by patients who have completed a good FIT training program are much more likely to be caused by insufficient adjustment to the realities of the disease than by ignorance. Mistakes due to inadequate information processing do occur, however. The following list includes the most frequent errors:

- **Underestimation of the Speed of Carbohydrate Absorption**

Many patients do not realize that if they do not increase the speed of absorption of preprandially injected regular insulin, the ideal interval between injecting and eating would be at least 45 minutes or more (Lean et al. 1985; Dimitriadis 1983). Since such a long interval is often impracticable, the only other possibility is to facilitate insulin absorption, especially when rapidly-absorbed carbohydrates are eaten.

- **Faulty Choice of Blood Glucose Target Points for Constant Corrections of Blood Glucose**

Due to poor predictability, postprandial corrections of hyperglycemic values are fairly risky. The relative risks of postprandial blood glucose corrections are multiplied if the correction aims at too low a target value, e.g., 100 mg/dl one hour after eating.

The preprandial target should never be lower than 100 mg/dl, except for certain pregnant and newly manifested patients. Patients often do not realize that the margin of error in self-monitoring can be be as large as 15–20 mg/dl, so that if they aim at 90 mg/dl, the value they achieve may actually be 70 mg/dl. An overdose of even one unit of insulin may thus lead to hypoglycemia in a relatively insulin-sensitive patient. After all, 70 minus 40 is 30. It must therefore be doubly emphasized that any blood glucose values under 90 mg/dl should be corrected upward (except in pregnancy). If this is neglected, the risk of hypoglycemia rises.

- **Eating While Hyperglycemic**

Lowering blood glucose, especially very high values (over 240 mg/dl) takes time. Many patients do not realize that if they eat in spite of hyperglycemia, blood glucose will decrease more slowly yet, even if a correction has been made. If the interval between consecutive corrections is too short (less than three hours), then sooner or later (probably later) hypoglycemia will follow. The mistake of eating while hyperglycemic might, therefore, simply be the result of a faulty estimate of the true degree of insulin deficit (although it can also take place for other reasons related to the Child ego state such as an inability to delay gratification – see also Sect. 13.3 below). At any rate, this is one of the most frequent mistakes made by patients.

- **Incorrect Algorithms**

Well-trained patients rarely make mistakes due to use of incorrect algorithms. When glycemic control improves, however, insulin sensitivity usually increases and insulin requirement falls. It is therefore important to take these potential changes into account, especially at the beginning of FIT. In our experience, the secondary adjustment of insulin dosage (correction of algorithms) needs to be given much more emphasis in the training program than the much simpler primary adjustment (correction of out-of-range blood glucose values).

13.3 Failure to Adjust to the Realities of Diabetes

Suboptimal adjustment to the reality of having diabetes almost always occurs when the Adult level is no longer responsible for controlling glycemia. Sect. 14.1, "Contraindications for functional insulin treatment," goes into this problem in detail. The diverse forms of denial manifest themselves most frequently through neglect of self-monitoring, poor record-keeping, and omitting prandial insulin injections. A classic example of denial of reality is the denial of the limits of insulin treatment in the sense that, "I can eat absolutely anything I want."

14 Frequent Physician-Related Problems

The most frequent physician-related problems can be classified in three categories:

1. Difficulties in communicating with patients;
2. Inability to understand what life is like for the patient;
3. Inadequate information.

14.1 Communication Problems

Training and motivating the patient for self-care have become essential components of the long-term treatment of chronic disease. Unfortunately, however, during the course of their medical studies few doctors learn how to teach patients at all, and even fewer learn how to teach in a group setting.

Many problems in communication stem from the physician's lack of knowledge about the stages the patient must work through in order to come to terms with his disease. A patient in the first stage of denial may be written off as being unreasonable; one who is working out his anger, as cantankerous; or one who is depressed, as impossible to motivate. Such problems of communication within the doctor-patient relationship can slow or even stop the patient's "grief-work" process.

Expressed in the terminology of transactional analysis, the problem is one of "crossed transactions." Instead of the Adult level, other levels of the patient's personality are addressed. Grief-work may be understood as the process of enabling the patient to react on the Adult level in order to work toward an optimum level of recovery. Addressing the patient on the Parent level (i.e., appealing to his internalized behavioral norms), for example, will not be very helpful because he is likely to respond on a Child level. In other words, presenting recommendations as a system of commands (e.g., "You must do this ...") and prohibitions (e.g., "Sweets are forbidden ...") is more likely to cause a desire to rebel than a wish to comply.

If the physician fails to recognize at what stage the patient is in his progress toward coming to terms with the disease, he may also fail to give adequate advice. For example, a patient who is denying reality may be planning a pregnancy or planning a risky job change in spite of proliferative retinopathy and approaching blindness. Such a patient needs directive counseling, which he may not receive if the physician does not realize what is going on. Denial of reality is a "normal" part of coming to terms with the disease, but this does not mean that it should be supported by the physician.

14.2 Inability to Understand What Life Is Like for the Patient

It is hardly possible to achieve consistently good metabolic control with current methods of insulin therapy unless the patient is able to correctly evaluate his glycemic level, inject insulin in any given social or psychological situation, and diagnose and immediately treat hypoglycemia on his own. This can only be feasible if the demands made on him are reduced to the bare essentials. What he is required to do must be as convenient as possible. This means that the physician or diabetes counselor must understand that certain compromises and accommodations are necessary, especially regarding blood glucose determination and techniques of insulin injection. For example, it would be impracticable to expect a person with a full-time job and an active social life to carry around a cumbersome glucose meter all day. If he is to make the frequent blood sugar measurements he needs to achieve good control (4–6 per day), probably 80% of them will have to be made without such a device. However, highly suitable, small blood glucose meters that measure very rapidly are now available. The situation is similar with insulin administration. For example, in Central Europe it is customary to eat 4–5 times per day (3 full meals, plus 1 or 2 snacks). To conform, the patient must make 6–7 insulin injections per day (one each time he eats plus two basal injections). **In any case, FIT cannot be carried out with less then 3 insulin injections per day.** So injection procedures must be as streamlined as possible. Insulin pens are a great help in this regard. **Procedures that are not abso lutely necessary** (such as keeping insulin refrigerated, disinfecting the injection site, changing needles for every injection) **must be omitted,** to make the therapy practicable enough for the patient to carry it out correctly on a long-term basis.

Near-normoglycemic metabolic control in type I (insulin-dependent) diabetes is practically impossible with current methods without taking some risk of hypoglycemia into the bargain. It is, therefore, absolutely necessary for the patient to carry glucose with him at all times. Here again, convenience is important, so a light, easily carried form of glucose should be chosen. Moreover, if patients report having no hypoglycemic episodes, the physician must be able to interpret this on the basis of HbA_{1c} and other clinical data. It usually means either that the patient has poor perception of hypoglycemic states, or that metabolic control is less than satisfactory.

A frequent mistake made by physicians is to attribute too low or too high blood glucose levels to the wrong causes and to suggest unnecessary algorithm modifications. Both hypoglycemic and hyperglycemic values are often simply the result of mistakes in dosage of prandial insulin. It is naive to believe that it is easy for the patient to correctly judge how much insulin he needs each time he eats. The physician needs to evaluate whether the patient needs more training in correct prandial insulin substitution before he recommends correcting the algorithms.

14.3 Inadequate Information

Actual deficits in the physician's knowledge are rare. Perhaps the area where the most mistakes are made is in insulin kinetics, especially the kinetics of delayed-acting insulins. For example, ultralente insulins have practically no peaks. Increasing or decreasing the morning or evening dose of an ultralente insulin will not influence a circumscribed part of the day; yet many physicians recommend doing so in order to correct high fasting blood glucose values. If blood sugar is high in the morning and nighttime hypoglycemia has been excluded, a differential diagnosis must be made between (a) insufficient overall basal insulinization and (b) the "dawn phenomenon," i.e., a relatively circumscribed early-morning increase in insulin requirement. If the "dawn phenomenon" is truly responsible, increasing the evening dose of ultralente insulin is effective only in exceptional cases. It would generally be better to change the type of basal insulin used from a long-acting ultralente to an intermediate NPH or lente insulin which should be injected late in the evening (see Sect. 5.1, "Basal substitution").

Another frequent mistake is to place too much importance on early postprandial blood glucose values (e.g., one hour after eating) when evaluating whether prandial substitution was appropriate.Early postprandial values give more information about whether the speed of insulin absorption matches that of carbohydrate absorption than about the suitability of the selected dose of insulin for the amount of carbohydrates consumed.

15 The "Contras"

15.1 Contraindications for Functional Insulin Treatment

Most patients who have been well-informed about FIT and who are undergoing a "normal" process of coming to terms with their diabetes would like to try FIT, unless they are committed to some other form of therapy and do not want to give it up. The only contraindications for FIT arise from an inability to carry it out; i.e., FIT is contraindicated if the patient is incapable of the required rational action. For example, small children and patients with psychiatric disorders (e.g., schizophrenics, patients with obsessive-compulsive neuroses, etc.) would not be suitable candidates for FIT. Patient do not have to be particularly brilliant to learn to carry out FIT, but with very low levels of intelligence would not be good candidates. Conditions such as depression, alcoholism, bulimia and anorexia can also severely restrict a persons ability to act rationally.

FIT cannot be carried out on a partial basis. If the patient is given the responsibility for his glycemic levels, then he must also have the opportunity and ability to make independent decisions about food intake and insulin dosage. In cases where the patient's ability to act rationally seems to be restricted, it is better to make a clear decision about whether he is capable of FIT or not, rather than to have him try only certain components.

Since the trainer's knowledge and experience ultimately determine the results both as to glycemic levels and risk to the patients, FIT should not be carried out unless experienced and knowledgeable therapists are available.

High risk of hypoglycemia is not a contraindication for FIT, but it is a contraindication for choosing a near-normoglycemic target range. History of hypoglycemia must be taken into account when choosing the target level for blood glucose and the algorithms for blood glucose correction (See Chap. 6, "Hypoglycemia").

15.2 "Difficult" Patients

The most difficult patients for a therapist to deal with are those who have not achieved an optimal adjustment to the realities of their disease. Within the framework of the theories on working through grief as well as transactional analysis, the phase of denial of reality should be differentiated from the depressive phase.

During the denial phase, it appears that the Child personality state dominates the patient's view of the world. His arguments against any rational suggestions offered by the therapist sound like a child's excuses to a parent. (For example, if he has been neglecting self-monitoring, "I can't do it during school... Anyway, it was only 110 when I got up... I really don't have time." If he is not keeping a self-monitoring record and his HbA_{1c} is high, "My blood sugar is good, anyway... Keeping records doesn't help... It's so boring!" Or if he has been omitting prandial insulin injections, "It was only one carbohydrate unit." He may also simply refuse to accept any of the treatment alternatives, i.e., either that eating anytime requires prandial insulin or that the continued hyperinsulinemia of conventional treatment requires planned food intake every three hours. Patients with more imagination may deny the predictability of blood glucose dynamics, "With me it's always different, no matter what I do." Or they may claim unusual consequences, "Yes, but my feet swell up when my blood sugar goes under 200... I just don't feel good when I'm below 150." It would be useless to try to argue with such patients on a rational level only. No amount of facts will convince them. They must first be helped to deal with their fears and anxieties before they can begin to accept reality.

It can be even harder to deal with patients who are in the depressive phase. According to Harris (1967), in depression there is an internal dialogue in which the Parent is "beating on the Child." When a rigid Parent predominates, the rules and prohibitions seem so overwhelming that any kind of action is precluded. Here again, rational arguments alone will be useless ("I just don't care") until the emotional aspects of the problem have been dealt with.

Another problematical type of patient is the perfectionist, who often shows obsessive-compulsive characteristics. For example, in spite of complete inability to recognize low blood sugar levels and/or in spite of approaching blindness, such patients may still insist on trying to maintain normoglycemia. Others may be extremely afraid of hypoglycemia ("I can't risk having others see me..."). In either case, the Parent, with its rules and prohibitions, seems to be the dominant factor. Here, too, the problem must be dealt with on an emotional rather than solely on a rational level.

The social environment in which the patient lives also plays a role in whether the Adult is free enough for rational action; for example, when there is a secondary gain associated with being sick (for example, a patient who faints only when her mother is around).

15.3 *Intermezzo 3:* A Strategy for Failure or How to Mess Things Up in the Outpatient Phase

Let us try to extend our ever expandable design for failure to the outpatient phase:

1. Take the danger of a patient's "libidinous attachment" to the doctor seriously. Make sure there are no opportunities for one to arise by having the patient see a different doctor at each clinic visit. It's always helpful to have only "brand new" colleagues do the counseling, so they can learn something from the patients.
2. In prescribing and proscribing, let yourself really go. Patients need to be bound by rules and regulations. Use the phrase, "You must..." as often as possible. Be sure to write down your orders for the insulin dosage algorithms so that the patient doesn't think about making any changes on his own.
   If the patient does come up with any individual practical suggestions or imaginative solutions to problems, be sure you don't take them seriously, or the patient might start getting ideas. Also, never explain the reasons for your orders, since the patient might say he doesn't think the situation was like that at all. He might even think he has a better solution.
3. Regard the patient who has completed a FIT training program as having learned all he can. He certainly wouldn't be capable of learning any more, so there is no use in trying to teach him. So don't bother evaluating his ability to deal with everyday problems. He wouldn't be able to improve, anyway. The outpatient visits should be dedicated to giving out rules and regulations, certainly not for further training or motivation.
4. Regard all patients as either "good" or "bad," and face the fact that people just can't change. If a bad patient does do something right, regard it as just a fluke. Lasting changes in motivation or behavior really aren't possible.
5. If a patient should have a hemoglobin A1c above normal, be sure to show him how displeased you are. Instead of calmly discussing the reasons with him, appeal to his conscience. Try to make him feel as guilty as possible. If he doesn't have a bad conscience (i.e., if his Parent isn't working overtime), he won't be motivated to change his behavior.
6. Don't worry that the patient might have anything else to do with his time besides busying himself with his diabetes. Be sure to show him how astonished you are if he doesn't manage to do the number of blood sugar determinations you told him were necessary. Always assume his actions are rational. If you should notice, for example, that a non-pregnant patient does at least 7–10 blood sugar tests a day or none at all, regard this as simply the way it is and don't bother about finding an explanation.
7. Recognize that a brittle diabetic patient is simply a brittle diabetic patient. Don't worry about trying to find the reasons for such wide swings in blood glucose. (By the way, if you place suitable emphasis on blood glucose values just above 220 and just below 60 mg/dl, you will be able to diagnose a large number of brittle diabetic patients.)

16 Checklist for Continuing Care of FIT Patients (Phase III of Rehabilitation)

Medical care, supervision, and counseling are just as important under FIT as in the long-term care of type I insulin-dependent diabetic patients under any type of therapy regime. The cooperation between patient and doctor is especially important in determining the long-term success in achieving good metabolic control (and thus in preventing late complications).

Through their interaction with the diabetic patient, physicians and diabetes counselors influence the following aspects of the disease and its treatment:

1. How much patients know about their disease and its treatment;
2. How well they can apply this knowledge, and whether therapy is practicable;
3. Their motivation;
4. Their ability to accept and come to terms with the disease;
5. Their metabolic status;
6. Late complications;
7. Other diseases they may have;
8. Their social environment;
9. Their contacts with the diabetes center;
10. Humor.

In striving to optimize the course of treatment, especially during phase III, the status of all of these points needs to be evaluated and, if necessary, improved. Aspects of points 1, 2 and 5 have already been discussed in Sect. 5.3, "Self-monitoring and Glycemic Control – Why Keep Records?"

16.1 The Patient's Knowledge

Optimal insulin substitution requires that the patient has enough theoretical knowledge to be able not simply to correct hyperglycemic values using fixed algorithms, but rather also to adjust the algorithms themselves to changes in insulin requirement.

It is therefore important to **check whether he correctly uses the algorithms** for basal and prandial insulin and for correcting out-of-range values (details are given in Chap. 5, "Criteria of Functional Insulin Treatment"), and **whether he is able to determine his actual total daily insulin requirement**. To do this, he must be able to analyze his records, comparing the total amou nt of insulin injected, total amount of carbohydrates consumed, and mean blood glucose (MBG). **If MBG rises above 160 (170) mg/dl or falls below 100 (110) mg/dl on three consecutive days, then he must realize that it is time to re-evaluate his algorithms (i.e., decide whether to make a secondary adjustment).**

The patient's general knowledge about diabetes (e.g., the significance of ketonuria and glucosuria, risks and prevention measures regarding late complications, etc.) should also be evaluated and updated from time to time.

If the patient's progress towards coming to terms with his disease is normal, the status of his knowledge should be under the control of the "data processing" system of his Adult personality state.

16.2 Applying Knowledge; Practicability of Therapeutic Measures

Good diabetes therapy should allow the patient to achieve the highest quality of life possible under the circumstances; i.e., disadvantages due to constantly having to take care of his diabetes should be prevented as far as possible. Compromises have to be made, however, since good metabolic control does require a fair amount of effort (sufficiently frequent self-monitoring, etc.). Applying knowledge to practice should ensure the maintenance of good metabolic control without severe acute complications (such as severe hypoglycemia) and without an unacceptable degree of effort.

The patient's ability to apply his knowledge to practice can be tested by checking whether he can determine, evaluate, and influence his blood sugar level in all kinds of situations; whether he can correctly modify his blood glucose target level as the situation requires; and whether he can administer insulin correctly and without complications, even in difficult situations. The frequency of hypoglycemic episodes can also be regarded as an indicator of his ability to apply his knowledge.

From the standpoint of transactional analysis, it can be said that application of knowledge involves cooperation between the Adult and Child personality levels. While the Adult is required for rational behavior, the Child contributes its drive toward autonomy and its joy in experimentation.

16.3 Motivation

Motivation can be divided into two components: intrinsic and extrinsic motivation (Diabetes Education Study Group 1985). Intrinsic motivation is determined by the individual's internal goals and priorities; it can also be described as the person's value system. Extrinsic motivation, on the other hand, comes from external factors and influences (e.g., social or material rewards). It is much less durable and therefore weaker than intrinsic motivation because it is only effective as long as the external pressure exists.

In terms of transactional analysis, something that is intrinsically motivating has inherent qualities that appeal to the Child ("It's fun... It makes me feel good to know I can do something well...") as well as to the rationality of the Adult. Extrinsic motivation relates more to the Parent's system of commandments and prohibitions ("My doctor said I should do this...")

How can motivation be increased? Positive reinforcement, i.e., ensuring that an act has positive (pleasant) consequences, is the most effective method, especially when the reinforcement is intrinsically motivating; e.g., when it simultaneously satisfies the Child's desire for fun and fulfills a rational (Adult) need. Positive social reinforcement – for example, praise – is an external influence, but when it satisfies the Child's need for affection and acceptance, it can also be very effective. So it would be useful for the diabetes counselor to ask himself the question, "How can I arrange things so that the treatment procedures are fun for the patient?" Or, "How can I praise the patient?"

International Study Group on Functional Insulin Treatment

PATIENT:
Name: Maria S.
Birth date: 1935 Tel.:
Address:
Diabetes since: 1974 Wt.: 66 kg

Functional insulin treatment (FIT) since ...

☒ with injections
○ with pump

INSULIN
- BASAL (fasting requirement): a.m. 11 UL / 1 REG U; p.m. 11 UL U
- PRANDIAL (meal-related): 1 CHO unit (12g) = 1 REG U
- Correction: 1 U regular ins. lowers my BG by approx. −40 mg/dl; 1 CHO unit (12 g carbohydrates) raises my BG by approx. +60 mg/dl

Target for correction of aberrant BG values
Fasting/pre-meal: 100 mg/dl (or ......)
After meals: 1 hour < 160 mg/dl (or < ......)
Target range for MBG: from ...... to ...... mg/dl

EXAMPLE: Diet (CHO units) ...
Insulin (U) ...

Date	TIME:	1 a.m.	2	3	4	5	6	7	8	9	10	11	12	1 p.m.	2	3	4	5	6	7	8	9	10	11	12	Total
Mon. 5/28	Delayed ins.	Ultralente						11														11				22 / 31
	Regular ins.							5						4												9
	BG							91			112			96						120				201		MBG 124
	CHO								3			1		4								1				9
	kcal								230			100		300								70				~700
Comments:																										
Tue. 5/29	Delayed ins.							11														11				22 / 30
	Regular ins.							3						5												8
	BG							107						111					145					234		MBG
	CHO								2					3								1				~6
	kcal								200					600								150				~900
Comments:																										
Wed.	Delayed ins.									11																
	Regular ins.									4																
	BG									96																MBG
	CHO									3																
	kcal																									
Comments:																										

Fig. 16.1. A somewhat overweight diabetic woman comes in for a check-up. She lives a long way from the treatment center.
What would you advise?
What questions would you ask her?

Apparently this patient regularly shows a decrease in blood glucose overnight. She has to go to bed with hyperglycemic values in order to wake up with normal values.

A reduction in basal insulin should be recommended (10-20% as a first step); i.e., new basal dose, 9–9 or 8–8 ultralente. Remember that even with a reducing diet, delayed-acting insulin should be less than 50% of total daily requirement. Changes in the dosage of regular insulin should only be considered after the basal insulin dose has been reduced.

The frequency of hypoglycemic episodes needs to be looked at any time that basal insulin makes up such a high proportion of total daily insulin dose. The risk of hypoglycemia is increased if the dose of delayed-acting insulin is (too) high.

In order to get the cooperation of the Adult, it helps to set concrete, realistic behavioral goals which can be reached within a short time. (The more immediate the positive reinforcement provided by reaching the goal, the more powerful its effects.) In our experience with FIT, trying to maintain motivation by means of commands and prohibitions (i. e., negative reinforcement such as, "You must keep your blood sugar down or you will develop late complications..." or "You cannot leave out an injection before a meal or your blood sugar will go sky high...") has been the least successful method.

16.4 Acceptance of Diabetes

The stages of grief work – denial of reality (domain of the Child), depression (domain of the Parent), and conscious acceptance of the disease (domain of the Adult) – have already been described in Chap. 13, "Frequent Patient-Related Problems." How can the process of coming to terms with diabetes be facilitated? This can probably be accomplished only by reinforcing the patient's autonomy and supporting rational action; i. e., from the standpoint of transactional analysis, appealing to the Adult personality level. Instead of commands and prohibitions, instead of prescribing behavior, when a problem arises it is more helpful to ask the patient, "What can we do about this particular problem?" or "What solutions would you suggest?"

16.5 Metabolic Status

The above-named factors, the patient's knowledge about his disease, ability to apply his knowledge, motivation, and acceptance of diabetes, all influence his metabolic status. Metabolic status should of course be monitored regularly by means of the usual parameters such as glycosylated hemoglobin, mean blood glucose, glucosuria, ketonuria, and body weight, plus the frequency of acute hypoglycemic or hyperglycemic complications.

16.6 Late Complications

The status regarding potential and/or already existing late complications should be checked at least once a year. In each individual case it is important to consider the statistical probability of microvascular complications (depending on duration of disease, level of glycemic control, and other risk factors such as cigarette smoking), what complications have already been diagnosed, and when they were last examined. It is absolutely necessary to inform patients about the risks of late complications, not as a tool for immediate motivation, but in a way that will help him to plan his future. It is not helpful, for example, to wait until creatinine reaches 6 mg/dl before educating the patient about kidney failure.

For patients who have already developed secondary hypertension, blood pressure reduction is even more important than normalizing blood sugar. There is evidence that the progression of renal complications (and also of retinopathy) can be slowed by a real near-normalization of blood pressure; i.e., to below 130 (or 120)/90 mmHg for younger diabetic patients. The conventional definition of hypertension is therefore no longer relevant here. The therapeutic goal must be considerably lower than usual and true physiological levels aimed for. For younger, relatively normal-weight diabetic patients, nonmedicationalmeasures such as restriction of dietary salt and weight loss have decreased in importance, since they are only rarely effective in this type of patient. Comprehensive patient education in the management of hypertension has proven invaluable in maintaining long-term normotensive blood pressure values in these patients (when microalbuminuria is elevated, at the latest). (An excellent example of such a program is one developed by Muehlhauser et al., 1986. See Table 16.1). In this model, training sessions are conducted weekly (total of 3–4 sessions). The program is based on the principles of self-monitoring of blood pressure and self-management of medication (whether ACE-inhibitors, cardioselective beta-blockers, diuretics, or vasodilators) under supervision of the physician.

Table 16.1. Summary of antihypertensive patient education program. Emphasis on secondary hypertension in diabetes mellitus.

Unit I:
- Definition and causes of hypertension (high blood pressure)
- Relation between diabetes mellitus and hypertension
- Detection of kidney damage in diabetes mellitus
- Antihypertensive treatment measures other than medication
- Stepwise plan for antihypertensive medication (outline)
- Self-monitoring of blood pressure

Unit II:
- Summary of factors leading to high blood pressure
- Significance of secondary hypertension in diabetes
- Frequent errors in measurement of blood pressure
- Types of medication and their characteristics
  - ACE-inhibitors
  - Ca-antagonists
  - beta-blockers
  - vasodilators
  - diuretics
- Discussion of self-monitored blood pressure records; adjustment of therapeutic measures

Unit III:
- Summary of antihypertensive medication
- Discussion of self-monitored blood pressure records; further adjustment of therapeutic measures
- Importance of antihypertensive therapy in prevention of late complications of diabetes
- Conditions for discontinuation of antihypertensive therapy
- Adjustment of therapy in a hypertensive crisis
- High blood pressure and other risk factors for coronary heart disease
- General discussion and summary

16.7 Comorbidity

Certain diseases may make it impossible for the patient to take responsibility for his actions, and thus impossible to carry out FIT (see Sect. 15.1, "Contraindications for functional insulin treatment"). This is the case, for example, with anorexia nervosa and bulimia. It is therefore important to diagnose and monitor the course of such illnesses, with particular attention to the consequences of any interactions with the diabetes. The therapy of any illness that diminishes the patient's autonomy and ability to act rationally should have a high priority.

16.8 Social Environment

Both the patient's occupational environment and the type and degree of interaction with his family and social circle can influence his metabolic control in many ways. Secondary gains from the role of "sick person" may effectively preclude attempts to achieve optimal control, for example. Lack of social integration may foster depression and the feeling that it is hopeless to try to improve metabolic control, besides preventing him from learning about new techniques and developments. **Self-help** groups can be immensely helpful in such situations. They have also proven extremely valuable in motivating patients and helping them to work through the process of accepting diabetes. In such cases they seem to take on the function of a catalyst in facilitating the process of coming to terms with the disease.

16.9 The Patient's Contact with the Diabetes Treatment Center, Physician or Diabetes Counselor

Just as the patient's role within the framework of FIT is different than it would be under conventional therapy, so also is the role of the physician. Under conventional therapy, the physician is responsible for the content of the patient's Parent level (behavioral norms); i.e., he is responsible for the patient's learning to say to himself, "I'm allowed to do this..., but I'm not allowed to do that...," or "I really should do..." Under FIT, the patient's Adult is the one who is responsible for glycemic control; for example, he might say to himself, "I can keep my blood sugar at my target level if I..." The task of the diabetes doctor or counselor is to help the patient to analyze and find solutions to the various problems that arise. Thus, his role is to facilitate the diabetes-related functioning of the patient's Adult (see also Sect. 16.3, "Motivation").

One of the most important aspects of the physician's his role is to help to maintain motivation. Here, it is important to facilitate optimal cooperation and balance between the patient's Child ("I wish..."), Adult ("How can I reach my goal?"), and Parent ("I should..."). For example, if the therapy goal is to achieve a near-normal HbA_{1c}, the doctor would want to motivate the patient to autonomous analysis of his records and regular contact with the diabetes center, since this will help improve HbA_{1c}. To keep the patient coming, he must especially try to appeal to the Child, for example, by giving the patient the feeling that there is always something new and interesting to learn at the visits.

16.10 Humor

"The great thing [about humor] apparently lies in the triumph of narcissism, in the victoriously asserted invulnerability of the ego. The ego refuses to be offended at the occasion provided by reality, to be obliged to suffer; it maintains its conviction that the traumas of the outside world cannot touch it, yes it even proves that they are only occasions for increasing pleasure." Thus did Freud describe the significance of humor in 1927, at about the same time that insulin was first being used in diabetes treatment. From the standpoint of transactional analysis, we might say that the great thing about humor lies in the victoriously asserted invulnerability of the **Child.**

Certainly diabetic patients waiting for dialysis or with rejected kidney transplants, or those in imminent danger of blindness, have little to laugh about. But their fate would surely be more bearable if they could be helped to laugh. Shouldn't this kind of aid also be a component of the physician's role?

17 Review of Results and Experience

A comprehensive description of all the data we have collected on the effectiveness of FIT training would be far beyond the scope of this book. A detailed analysis of our results – in regard to metabolic, psychological, and psychosocial variables – was published in monograph* form. The following analysis will restrict itself to the metabolic results achieved with the first group of 159 patients to complete the program. This original training program was carried out during the years 1983–1986 at the I. Medical Department of the University of Vienna Medical School. This program was carried out with hospitalized patients under conditions that were not particularly conducive to group patient education. The program was later moved to another facility of the University of Vienna Medical School (at the Department of Biomedical Engineering and Physics) and converted to an outpatient basis in which the phases can be carried out at different points in time (See also Chap. 2, "Overview of the Phases of Rehabilitation..."). On the basis of these later experiences, we have come to following conclusions:

- Outpatient education is much cheaper and equally effective;
- With adequate supervision, the frequency of severe acute complications with outpatient training is negligible;
- Patient acceptance is greater with outpatient training;
- Most importantly, outpatient training allows a modular structure in which the tempo of overall rehabilitation and the goals, content and time points of the training program can be adapted to individual needs while retaining a group structure. This makes it possible to maintain high standards with a relatively small staff.

---

* Howorka, Thesis for degree in Hospital management (1994): Quality assurance in treatment and rehabilitation of diabetes mellitus

17.1 Patients

Beginning with the establishment of the first training program in April 1983, up to January 1986, a total of 159 consecutive, unselected patients were trained in FIT. Follow-up examinations were conducted on 146 patients. The mean age was 29 yrs ± 11 yrs (± SD); range 12–64 yrs. The mean duration of diabetes was 11 ± 7 (0–46) yrs; 63% of the patients were women. Late complications were present in 65%. One patient was completely blind, two were partially blind. Four patients were undergoing chronic dialysis (two received successful kidney transplants, success being achieved for one on the second try).

Only 20% of patients had received any formal diabetes education before beginning FIT, and only six had completed a comprehensive diabetes education program (Mühlhauser et al. 1983).

All socioeconomic levels were represented. Seven patients were unemployed, four were in prison, the rest were employed in various occupations. Two-thirds of the patients had been labeled "brittle diabetics" by other hospitals.

17.2 Follow-up

Patients from the Vienna metropolitan area were usually seen in the department's outpatient clinic approx. every two months after completing the training program. Patients who lived at greater distances were seen every six months. The mean interval between completion of the program and the follow-up visit used for this analysis was 16 ± 8 months (146 patients). During this period a mean of 8 ± 7 (median, 6) outpatient visits had been completed (during pregnancies, patients made weekly visits).

Hemoglobin A_{1c} was determined using microcolumn chromatography (Biorad, Richmond, U.S.A.). Blood and urine glucose were determined at the follow-up visits using the hexokinase method, and other routine examinations (blood lipids, kidney function, etc.) were carried out according to standard procedures.

Prospective analyses of data from follow-up visits as well as patient diaries (blood glucose, insulin dosage, and nutrient intake) were made with computer support (Czerwenka-Howorka 1984c). The significance of differences over time was tested using paired t-tests or the Wilcoxon test.

A standardized questionnaire concerning frequency of acute complications, blood glucose self-measurements and insulin injections as well as various aspects of the practicability of FIT was completed by all patients after one year of experience with FIT.

17.3 Results

17.3.1 Acceptance of FIT

Of 162 patients originally offered the opportunity for FIT training, only three refused even to try. Of the 159 patients who underwent training, two preferred to return to their previous regime of two injections per day. Of the remaining 157 patients, 16 were eventually judged by the therapist to be incapable of carrying out FIT correctly, although they wished to continue FIT. The major reasons for incapability were of a psychological nature (e.g., severe depression, anorexia and/or bulimia, alcoholism) or were due to problems in the social environment (prison, delinquency due to neglect, etc.).

17.3.2 Metabolic Control

During the cumulative observation period of 190 patient-years, there was a decrease in mean blood glucose (mg/dl) from 197 ± 63 ($X \pm SD$; median, 196) before the start of FIT training to 132 ± 26 during the observation period, and 139 ± 44 (median, 131) at the end of the observation period; $p < 0.0001$). HbA_{1c} (%) decreased from 7.7 ± 1.7 (median, 7.5) to 6.3 ± 1.2; (median, 6.0) during, and 6.3 ± 1.5 (median, 6.1) at the end of the observation period (see Fig. 17.1).

The following factors were related to level of metabolic control under FIT: initial level of HbA_{1c}, frequency of self-monitoring and diary keeping; frequency of outpatient visits; age (i.e., adolescents showed the poorest metabolic control); and insulin requirement (patients requiring more than 60 IU/day showed the poorest control).

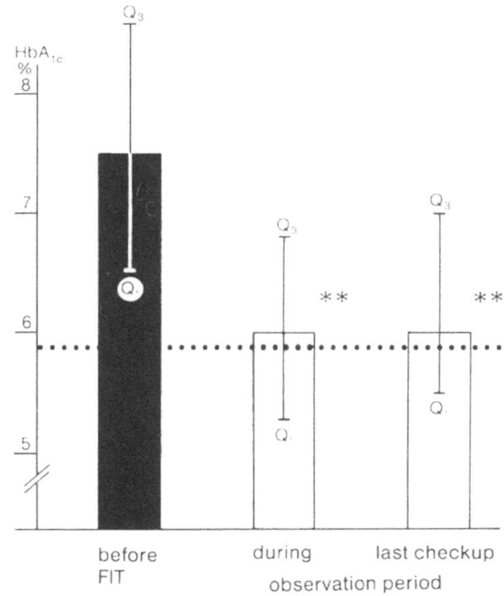

Fig. 17.1. HbA_{1c} in 146 unselected patients with type I (insulin-dependent) diabetes before, during, and at the last checkup of the observation period of 16 ± 8 months (Median; Q1-Q3), $**p < 0.0001$ vs. conventional treatment.

17.3.3 Acute Complications

Mild hypoglycemia occurred with a frequency of 1.3 episodes per week. The incidence of severe hypoglycemic attacks with loss of consciousness was 0.3 (1995: 0.21) episodes per patient-year; however, severe hypoglycemia occurred in only 12% of patients. The prophylactic measures described in Chap. 6, "Hypoglycemia," became routine and the incidence of severe hypoglycemia decreased after the introduction of these measures.

In spite of the fact that patients were recommended not to disinfect the injection site and that each injection needle was used at least several times, no cases of cutaneous complications were seen. (The total number of skin pricks, including both for self-monitoring of BG and for insulin administration, during the cumulative observation period of 190 patient-years was estimated to be over one million.) There were also no episodes of ketoacidosis requiring hospitalization.

17.4 Experience with FIT in Special Situations

Blindness: Blind patients can carry out FIT without difficulty, provided they have a suitable insulin pen or infusion device, plus help with self-monitoring.

Pumps: Only 5% of FIT patients preferred to administer insulin with a subcutaneous insulin infusion device rather than multiple daily injections.

Hemodialysis: Experiences with uremic patients who were undergoing hemodialysis were very positive. Since insulin requirement varies widely under hemodialysis, FIT would seem to be practically the only possible way to achieve good control. Patients trained in our program were also able to successfully manage insulin substitution almost without help during the extremely difficult transition phase after kidney transplantation.

Pregnancy: Diabetes-related complications during pregnancy were practically eliminated in our FIT patients (Howorka et al. 1996). The basis for this is preconceptional training of the patient in FIT. If a woman came to us after the beginning of pregnancy, a two-step procedure was used:

1. Immediate initial intervention (phase 0 and phase I): intensive diabetes education over 4–5 days, similar to the model described by Berger et al. (1983a).
2. Complete FIT group training program (phase II) at the earliest possible date (Howorka et al. 1996).

Psychosocial problems: As previously mentioned, the poorest results were obtained for patients who had severe psychological or social problems (delinquency, prison, behavioral disorders, bulimia, etc.). It must therefore be emphasized that if FIT is to be attempted with such patients, it should only be used in conjunction with, never instead of, proper psychosocial reintegrative measures.

18 Open Questions, Unsolved Problems and Limits of FIT

If delayed-acting insulin is injected twice daily, either NPH, lente or ultralente insulins can be used for basal substitution. We have also studied proinsulin in an intraindividual comparative study and found it to be very well-suited for this purpose. Unfortunately, the production of proinsulin was discontinued. Its controversial cardiovascular side effects have never been investigated under controlled conditions in type I diabetic patients.

The optimal route of delivery for prandial insulin is open. It is clear, however, that if CSII is used, prandial insulin should be delivered in the form of a bolus, rather than a rectangular profile (Sonnenberg 1983). The advantages of intramuscular or even intravenous administration of regular insulin with multiple injections have not been sufficiently examined. Rapidly absorbable insulin analogues should prove their advantages in the near future.

Prandial insulin requirement appears to be determined not only by the amount of carbohydrates consumed, but also to a certain extent by fat and protein. Hitherto existing data regarding the modification of insulin dosage in relation to type and degree of refinement of carbohydrates as well as amount of non-carbohydrates have been strictly empirical and should be more systematically investigated.

Rules of thumb have been formulated for the correction of off-target blood glucose values, but the expected drop in blood glucose produced by administration of regular insulin under basal conditions has not been systematically investigated. The rules for algorithm correction are therefore based on patient reports of their experience.

The limits of FIT arise from the conditions required to achieve optimal insulin substitution:

- Proper training and continued cooperation of patients is absolutely essential for carrying out FIT, but without a trained therapist, it is impossible to train and motivate patients. This can be a serious problem, especially in countries where the health system is publicly financed and an out-of-date bureaucracy does not recognize the need for diabetes educators.
- Intensive group instruction followed by individual counseling lays the foundation for a productive relationship between the chronically ill patient and his physician. In most countries, however, doctors learn little or nothing in medical school about what should be taught, how to teach, how to communicate with patients, or how to facilitate motivation for self-management of therapy. Even today, (group) patient education is often still considered unscientific, unnecessary, or even a hindrance to existing rigid concepts of the doctor-patient relationship.
- The correct estimation of carbohydrate intake and the corresponding prandial insulin requirement form the basis of decisions as to insulin dosage, but this is an area where patients frequently make mistakes. Unfortunately, currently available training techniques are not very effective.
- Efforts to achieve normoglycemic control are presently restricted primarily by the risk of hypoglycemia. Prediction of when it will occur and detection of its onset in time to prevent it are only possible in a very limited degree. The development of some sort of biological sensor would be of enormous help, especially for patients with impaired awareness of hypoglycemia.

Near-normoglycemia seems to have been finally accepted in most European countries as the goal of treatment for Type I (insulin-dependent) diabetes mellitus (Hanssen et al. 1986; Mühlhauser et al. 1987). The Diabetes Complication and Control Trial (DCCT Research Group 1987, 1990) will presumably provide hard evidence on points that are still controversial. Even if the issue of near-normoglycemia is not completely resolved, more and more diabetologists appear to agree that improving the diabetic patient's quality of life – and freeing him from a regimented diet and resulting behavioral restrictions – is an equally important therapeutic goal.

19 Epilogue

In the history of clinical diabetes there have never been so many unequivocal indications of the decisive importance of patient education for public health as there are at present (Assal et al. 1985). Unfortunately, however, there still appear to be serious obstacles to training insulin-treated diabetic patients to manage their own insulin therapy.

For understandable, but mainly historical reasons with little relevance to present need, the established structure of the health system in many parts of the world emphasizes "acute" medicine, mainly in the form of pharmacological crisis intervention in hospitalized patients. In the field of diabetes, preventive medicine - whether measures for preventing metabolic crises or preventing catastrophe caused by late complications - receives lip service, but is widely neglected in practice. Unfortunately, systematic, structured patient education programs are still such a novelty that integrating them into hospital routine usually requires far-reaching restructuring of personnel, space and organization. The necessity for training physicians and paramedical personnel in pedagogical aspects of patient education is often simply ignored.

Interdisciplinary cooperation between health educators, physicians, nurses, dietitians, psychologists and social workers would best fulfill the psychosocial, pedagogical and pharmacotherapeutic requirements for long-term care of the chronically ill. Only rarely do medical schools teach their students how to work in an interdisciplinary team as equal partners with a clear division of responsibility to pursue the goal of continuing education and motivation of the patient for self-management of therapy.

Furthermore, educating patients involves unforeseeable dynamic processes that can change the doctor-patient relationship in a way that may not be very comfortable from the doctor's point of view. Being pushed off a traditional pedestal and "degraded" to an equal partner (who can be chosen – or not – by the well-informed patient) cannot be an easy situation to deal with.

In a doctor's practice, and even in a diabetes center, the status of patient education and counseling is often determined by immediate considerations of economy. To prescribe insulin twice daily takes about 4 minutes. To train a patient in functional insulin substitution (phase 0–phase 2) takes at least 500 times as long. Moreover, traditional attitudes to various aspects of diabetes are now often a hindrance to progress. For example, mild hyperglycemia is usually accepted in practice as inevitable, and certainly less troublesome than hypoglycemia, which, as a complication caused by the treatment itself, is an understandable embarrassment to the doctor. Add to this the common judgment of "patient not motivated," and an increase in the entropy of the system is certain.

I sincerely hope that creative solutions to these problems can be found, perhaps outside the traditional framework of hospital care. Even if it were true that patient education brings no financial, institutional, or academic benefits, it does have one enormous advantage that outweighs all its disadvantages: the gratitude of the patients.

In the foreword to this book, FIT was called a rational therapy. This is true, but if I have succeeded in showing that there are also intuitive-emotional grounds for choosing, applying or advocating FIT, then I will feel that the goal of this book has been reached. Wide-ranging liberation from therapy-related restrictions, a quality of life undiminished by prohibition of spontaneity, and active self-responsibility in carrying out therapy – all continually gain in importance in the long-term care of insulin-treated diabetic patients. It is the balanced, pragmatic combination of emotions and intellect that leads to therapeutic success under FIT, but only if the physician/counselor recognizes and accepts the importance of these motivational factors, takes them into consideration, and bolsters them with suitable knowledge and action.

Whoever is pursuing similar goals and using similar standards in the long-term care of the chronically ill would be able to help to improve the FIT approach by contributing his experience and, perhaps, better solutions to individual problems as well as ways of adapting FIT to conditions in different localities. The first successes with FIT led to the founding of an Austrian "Working Group for Diabetes Education and Functional Insulin Treatment" in 1986, in Vienna, and to the establishment of an annual international training seminar for physicians and diabetes educators in functional insulin treatment. The goal is to spread the method while maintaining high standards of quality. The "International Study Group for Diabetes Education and Functional Insulin Therapy," which was founded by the graduates of the first training seminars, set the same goals for itself. The special advantage of such an international group is the standardized documentation of patient data, record forms, etc., which makes centralized analysis and international comparison possible. A recent survey of this group shows that at least several thousand insulin-treated diabetic patients in several countries have already been trained in functional insulin treatment.

I sincerely hope that you, the reader of this book, will keep me informed about your own ideas and experiences, so that hopefully future editions of this book will serve our common goals even more usefully.

The logo of the Study Group on Functional Insulin Substitution is the seagull, symbolizing our hopes that, just as for Jonathan Livingston Seagull, our diabetic patients will be able to regain their freedom to live a full and almost unrestricted life.

Vienna, Summer 1995 *Kinga Howorka*

Acknowledgments:
I wish to thank the many people who were instrumental in the development and methodological improvements in FIT. My deepest gratitude goes to the patients themselves, without whose experiences, creativity and cooperation, FIT would not have developed into its present form. The cooperation and enthusiasm of the patients was invaluable in overcoming many of the obstacles that originally stood in the way of establishing a structured patient education program, so that diabetes education is gradually becoming a matter of course in Austria.

I received help in writing this book from many quarters. I especially want to thank Prof. Dr. Herwig Thoma, Dr. Helga Grillmayr, Prof. Dr. Michael Berger, and Dr. Viktor Joergens for constructive criticism of the manuscript. I also wish to thank Dr. Ingrid Mühlhauser, Dr. Monika Grüsser, Ms. Gertrude Reiss, Dr. Michael Kroetlinger, Dr. Michael Jonas, Dr. Peter Damjancic, Ms. Ingeborg Kupfer, Mag. phil. Adam Jaworski, Dozent Dr. Josef Egger, Prof. Dipl. Ing. Dr. Rudolf

Dutter, Prof. Dr. Werner Waldhäusl and Prof. Dr. Dr. h.c. Erwin Deutsch for their invaluable advice. I also wish to thank Dipl.-Dolm. Irene Lehfuss-Brodnig for her untiring aid in preparation of the manuscript. I am extremely grateful to Dr. Jay Skyler for his help in editing the book.

I wish to express my **deepest gratitude** to Kathryn Nelson, who took on the horrendous task of adapting the 4th German edition of this book and transferring the ideology of FIT into English We both warmly thank our families, especially the fathers of our small children, for their patience, support, babysitting abilities, and (almost) never-ending tolerance.

References

Arbeitsgemeinschaft Diabetikerschulung: Arbeitsunterlage Typ I Diabetikerschulung. (Ed.: Österreichische Diabetesgesellschaft) 1985

Assal J.P., Pernet A.: Education as a part of therapy. In: World book of diabetes in practice. (Ed.: Krall L.P.) Exerpta Medica, 73–78, Amsterdam, 1982

Assal J.P., Mühlhauser I., Pernet A., Berger M.: Patient education as the basis for diabetes care in clinical practice and research. Diabetologia 28: 602–613, 1985

Berger M., Berchtold P., Cüppers H.J., Drost H., Kley H.K., Müller W.A., Wregelmann W., Zimmermann-Telschow H., Gries F.A., Krüskemper H.L., Zimmermann H.: Metabolic and hormonal effects of muscular exercise in juvenile type diabetics. Diabetologia 13: 355–365, 1977

Berger M., Cüppers H.J., Chantelau E.A., Sonnenberg G., Jörgens V.: Absorption kinetics of subcutaneously injected insulin preparations. In: Insulin update 1982 (Ed.: Skyler J.S.), Exerpta Medica, 97–110, Amsterdam, Genf, 1982

Berger M., Jörgens V., et al.: Praxis der Insulintherapie. Springer Verlag, Berlin, Heidelberg, 1983 (1986 2. Edition)

Berger M., Jörgens V., Mühlhauser I., Zimmermann H.: Die Bedeutung der Diabetikerschulung in der Therapie des Typ I Diabetes. Dtsch. Med. Wschr. 11: 424–430, 1983

Berne E.: Transactional analysis in psychotherapy. Grove Press, New York, 1961

Bernstein R.K.: Diabetes: The glucograf method for normalizing blood sugar. Crown Publ. Inc., New York, 1981

Besser-Siegmund C.: Easy weight. Econ Publishers, Düsseldorf, 2. edition, 1992

Bolli G.B., Gerich J.: The "dawn phenomenon" – a common occurence in both non-insulin-dependent and insulin-dependend diabetes mellitus. New Engl. J. Med. 310: 746–750, 1984

Bottermann P., Wahl K., Ermler R., Lebender A., Gyaram H.: Action profiles and plasma concentrations of insulin after s.c. application of different insulin preparations. In: Computer systems for insulin adjustment in diabetes mellitus, (Eds.: Beyer J., Albisser M., Schrezenmeir J., Lehmann L.), 85–109, Panscienta Verlag, Hedingen, 1985

Brange J., Skelbaek-Pedersen B., Langkjaer L., Damgaard U., Ege H., Havelund S., Heding L.G., Jorgensen K.H., Lykkeberg J., Markussen J., Pingel M., Rasmussen E.: Galenics of insulin preparations. In: Subcutaneous Insulin Therapy (Ed.: Berger M.), Springer-Verlag, Berlin-Heidelberg-New York, 1987

Bruns W., Bombor H., Jutzi E., Ratzmann K.P., Schulz B., Abel P., Fischer U.: Reproducibility of insulin dosage on consecutive days of blood glucose control by an artificial beta-cell in brittle diabetic patients. Diabetes Care 6: 112–117, 1983

Campbell P.J., Bolli G.B., Cryer P.E., Gerich J.E.: Pathogenesis of the dawn-phenomenon in patients with insulin-dependent diabetes mellitus. New Engl. J. Med. 312: 1473–1479, 1985

Chantelau E., Sonnenberg G.E., Stanitzek-Schmidt I., Best F., Altenähr H., Berger M.: Diet liberalization and metabolic control in Type I diabetic outpatients treated by continuous subcutaneous insulin infusion. Diabetes Care 5: 612–616, 1982

Chantelau E., Berger M.: Neue Aspekte zur Diät bei Typ I Diabetes mellitus. Dtsch. Med. Wschr. 110: 71–75, 1985

Chantelau E.A., Spraul M., Gösseringer G.: Alkohol und Typ I Diabetes mellitus. Dtsch. Med. Wschr. 110: 1393–1394, 1985

Constam G.R., Berger W.: Leitfaden für Zuckerkranke. Schwabe & Co. AG Verlag, Basel - Stuttgart, (10. Auflage), 1985

Coustan D.R., Reece E.A., Sherwin R.S., Rudolf M.C.J., Bates S.E., Sockin S.M., Holford T., Tamborlane W.V.: A randomized clinical trial of the insulin pump vs intensive conventional therapy in diabetic pregnancies. JAMA 5: 631–636, 1986

Cranston I., Lomas J., Maran A., Macdonald I., Amiel S.A.: Restoration of hypoglycaemia awareness in patients with long duration of insulin-dependent diabetes. Lancet 344: 283–879, 1994

Czerwenka-Howorka K., Bratusch-Marrain P., Waldhäusl W.: Algorithmen der normoglykämischen Insulinsubstitution bei Typ I Diabetes: Erste Langzeitergebnisse. Wiener klinische Wochenschrift 14: 558–559, 1984

Czerwenka-Howorka K., Waldhäusl W.: Optimized normoglycemic insulin replacement by a pen-shaped regular insulin delivery device. Life Support Systems, 2 (Suppl. 1): 24–26, 1984

Czerwenka-Howorka K., Gring H., Dorda W., Derfler K., Waldhäusl W.: Computerunterstützte Erfassung der Therapieeffizienz bei Diabetes mellitus. In: Medizinische Informatik 84 (Hrsg: Gell G., Eichtinger C.): 157–162, Verlag Oldenburg, Wien, München, 1984

Czerwenka-Howorka K., Waldhäusl W.: Verminderung der Hypo- und Hyperglykämieexposition bei Typ I Diabetes: Algorithmen der nahe-normoglykämischen Insulinsubstitution (NIS), Klinische Wochenschrift 109 (Suppl. IV): 44, 1985

de Shazer S.: Clues, investigating solutions in brief therapy. Norton Publ. New York 1988

DCCT Research Group: Diabetes Control and Complications Trial (DCCT): Results of Feasibility Study. Diabetes Care 10: 1–19, 1987

DCCT Research Group: Diabetes Control and Complications Trial (DCCT): Update, Diabetes Care 13: 427–433, 1990

DCCT Research Group: Epidemiology of severe hypoglycaemia in the diabetes control and complications trial. Am J Med 90: 450–9, 1991

DCCT Research Group: The effect of intensive treatment of diabetes on the development and progression of long-term complications in insulin-dependent diabetes mellitus. N Engl J Med 32: 971–86, 1993
Diabetes Education Study Group of the European Association for the Study of Diabetes: Motivating the diabetic patient. In: The Teaching Letter, (Eds.: Assal J.Ph., Liniger C.), 37–40, Genf, 1985
Dimitriadis G.D., Gerich J.E.: Importance of timing of preprandial subcutaneous insulin administration in the management of diabetes mellitus. Diabetes Care 6: 374–377, 1983
Egger H.: ALG-NIS: Ein Programm zur Berechnung patientenspezifischer Algorithmen für die nahe-normoglykämische Insulinsubstitution (NIS). Diplomarbeit am Institut für Statistik und Wahrscheinlichkeitstheorie, Abteilung für Technische Statistik der Technischen Universität Wien, 1986
Fanelli C., Epifano L., Rambotti A.M. et al: Meticulous prevention of hypoglycaemia (near-) normalizes magnitude and glycaemic thresholds of neuroendocrine responses to, symptoms of, and cognitive function during hypoglycaemia in intensively treated patient with IDDM of short duration. Diabetes 42: 1683–9, 1993
Fanelli C., Pampanelli S., Epifano L., Rambotti A.M., Di Vicenco A. et al: Long-term recovery from unawareness, deficient counterregulation and lack of cognitive dysfunction during hypoglycaemia, following institution of rational, intensive insulin therapy in IDDM. Diabetologia 37: 1265–76, 1994
Field J.B., Williams H.E., Mortimore G.E.: Studies on the mechanism of ethanol-induced hypoglycemia. J. Clin. Invest. 42: 497–505, 1963
Freud S.: Der Humor (1927) In: Sigmund Freud, Studienausgabe Band IV, Fischer Verlag, Frankfurt/Main, 1970
Freud S.: Trauer und Melancholie (1914/1917) In: Sigmund Freud, Studienausgabe Band III: Psychologie des Unbewußten, Fischer Taschenbuch Verlag, Frankfurt/Main, 1982
Fuhrmann K., Reiher H., Semmler K., Fischer F., Fischer M., Glöckner E.: Prevention of congenital malformations in infants of insulin-dependent diabetic mothers. Diabetes Care 3: 219–223, 1983
Galloway J.A.: New directions in drug development: mixtures, analogues, and modeling. Diab Care 16, Suppl. 3: 16–23, 1993
Gfeller R., Assal J.Ph.: Das Krankheitserlebnis des Diabetespatienten. Folia psychopractica 10, (Eds.: Hoffmann-LaRoche & Co. AG), Basel, 1979
Grinder J., Bandler R.: The structure of magic. Science and behaviour books, Inc., Palo Alto, 1976
van Halle B., Slama G., Pehuet M., Soria J., Predine J., Klein J.C., Tchobroutsky G.: Closed-loop evaluation of circadian insulin requirements (basal needs) in insulin-dependent diabetics. In: New approaches to insulin therapy, (Eds.: Irsigler K., Kunz K., Owens D.R., Regal H.), 169–170, MTP Press Limited, Lancaster, 1981
Hanssen K.F., Dahl-Jörgensen K., Lauritzen T., Feldt-Rasmussen B., Brinchmann-Hansen O., Deckert T.: Diabetic control and microvascular complications: The near-normoglycaemic experience. Diabetologia 29: 677–684, 1986

Harris T.A.: I'm o.k. – You're o.k.: A practical guide to transactional analysis. Harper & Row, New York, 1967

Harris A. Bjork, Harris T.A.: Staying OK. Harper & Row, New York, 1985

Holmes C.S., Hayford J.T., Gonzalez J.L., Weydert J.A.: A survey of cognitive functioning at different glucose levels in diabetic persons. Diabetes Care 6: 180–185, 1983

Howorka K.: Insulin-dependent? The functional use of insulin. Patient's handbook. Kirchheim Publishers, Mainz 1987 (1995 5th german edition)

Howorka K.: Quality assurance in treatment and rehabilitation of diabetes mellitus. Thesis for degree in Hospital Management (Univ. of Economy, Vienna) 1994

Howorka K., Heger G., Schabmann A., Anderer P., Tribl G., Zeitlhofer J: Hypoglycaemia unawareness in diabetes is associated with an early decrease in vigilance during hypoglycaemia. Psychoneuroendocrinology, 21, 1996 (in press)

Howorka K., Pumprla J., Feiks A., Schlusche C., Nowotny C., Ulm M., Schober E.: Modular education for diabetes and pregnancy: outcome analysis in 58 diabetic pregnancies under functional insulin treatment. Geburtshilfe und Frauenheilkunde, 1996 (in press)

Jenkins D.J.A., Taylor R.H., Wolever T.M.S.: The diabetic diet, dietary carbohydrate and differences in digestibility. Diabetologia 23: 477–484, 1982

Joslin E.P.: Diabetic Manual (3rd edition, Lea & Febiger) Philadelphia, New York, 1924

Jovanovic L., Peterson C.M.: Management of the pregnant, insulin-dependent diabetic woman. Diabetes Care 1: 63–68, 1980

Kemmer F.W., Berchtold D., Berger M., Starke A., Cüppers H.J., Gries F.A., Zimmermann H.: Exercise induced fall of blood glucose in insulin-treated diabetics unrelated to alteration of insulin mobilization. Diabetes 28: 1131–1137, 1980

Kübler-Ross E.: On death and dying. Macmillan Comp., New York, 1969

Kunze M., Exel W., Schoberberger R.: Schlank ohne Diät, 6th edn. Orac Verlag, Vienna, 1991

Lean M.E.J., Ng L.L., Tennison B.R.: Interval between insulin injection and eating in relation to blood glucose control in adult diabetics. Brit. Med. J. 290: 105–108, 1985

Lindsay A.N., Hardy S., Jarrett L., Rallison M.L.: High-carbohydrate, high fibre diet in children with Type I diabetes mellitus. Diabetes Care 7: 63–74, 1984

Miller E., Hare J.W., Cloherty J.P., Dunn P.J., Gleason R.E., Soeldner J.S., Kitzmiller J.L.: Elevated maternal hemoglobin A1c in early pregnancy and major congenital anomalies in infants of diabetic mothers. New Engl. J. Med. 304: 1331–1333, 1981

Mühlhauser I., Schernthaner G.: Diabetikerschulung mit dem Ziel der Selbsttherapie – Grundlage jeder erfolgreichen Diabetesbehandlung. Österr. Ärztezeitung 37: 263–267, 1982

Mühlhauser I., Jörgens V., Berger M., Graninger W., Gürtler W., Hornke L., Kunz A., Schernthaner G., Scholz V., Voss H.E.: Bicentric evaluation of a teaching and treatment programme for Type I (insulin-dependent) diabetic patients: Improvement of metabolic control and other measures of diabetes care for up to 22 months. Diabetologia 25: 470–476, 1983

Mühlhauser I., Broermann Ch., Bartels Ch., Bartels H., Berg R., Schwarz S., Berger M.: Qualitätskontrolle der Blutzucker-Selbstmessung bei unausgewählten Typ I Diabetikern. Bedeutung der Patientenschulung. Dtsch. Med. Wschr. 109: 1553-1557, 1984

Mühlhauser I., Sawicki P.: Wie behandle ich meinen Bluthochdruck. Blutdruckselbstmessung, Ernährung, Medikamente. Kirchheim-Verlag, Mainz, 1986

Mühlhauser I., Bruckner J., Howorka K.: Near-normoglycaemia and microvascular complications. Diabetologia 30: 47-48, 1987 (Letter)

Nuttall F.Q.: Diet and the diabetic patient. Diabetes Care 6: 197-207, 1983

Oyen D., Chantelau E.A., Berger M.: Zur Geschichte der Diabetesdiät. Springer Verlag Berlin-Heidelberg-New York-Tokyo, 1985

Perriello G., De Feo P., Torlone E., Fanelli C., Santeusanio F., Brunetti P., Bolli G.B.: The dawn phenomenon in Type 1 (insulin-dependent) diabetes mellitus: magnitude, frequency, variability and dependency on glucose counterregulation and insulin sensitivity. Diabetologia 34: 21-28, 1991

Phillips M., Simpson R.W., Holmann R.R., Turner R.C.: A simple and rational twice daily insulin regime. Distinction between basal and meal insulin requirements. Quart. J. Med. 191: 493-506, 1979

Pramming S., Thorsteinson B., Thailgaard A., Pinner E.M., Binder C.: Cognitive function during hypoglycaemia in Type 1 diabetes mellitus. Brit. Med. J. 229: 647-650, 1986

Reeves M.L., Seigler D.E., Ryan E.A., Skyler J.S.: Glycemic control in insulin-dependent diabetes mellitus. Comparison of outpatient intensified conventional therapy with continuous insulin infusion. Am. J. Med. 72: 673-680, 1982

Rizza R.A., Gerich J.E., Haymond M.W., Westland B.A., Hall L.D., Clemens A.H., Service F.J.: Control of blood sugar in insulin-dependent diabetes: Comparison of an artificial endocrine pancreas, continuous subcutaneous insulin infusion and intensified conventional insulin therapy. New Engl. J. Med. 303: 1313-1318, 1980

Schade D.S., Santiago J.V., Skyler J.S., Rizza R.A.: Intensive Insulin Therapy, Excerpta Medica, Amsterdam, 1983

Schade D.S., Argound G.M.: Subcutaneous versus intravenous insulin: The hypoglycaemic profiles of bolus injections. In: Clinical experiences with NovoPen. Proceedings of the Third International Hvidore Symposium: 25-28, 1985

Schiffrin A., Belmonte M.: Multiple daily self glucose monitoring: Its essential role in long term glucose control in insulin-dependent diabetic patients treated with pump and multiple subcutaneous injections. Diabetes Care 5: 479-484, 1982

Schiffrin A., Belmonte M.M.: Comparison between continuous subcutaneous insulin infusion and multiple injections of insulin. A one year prospective study. Diabetes 31: 255-264, 1982

Schiffrin A., Desrosiers M., Belmonte M.: Evaluation of two methods of self blood glucose monitoring by trained insulin-dependent diabetic adolescents outside the hospital. Diabetes Care 6: 166-169, 1983

Schiffrin A., Parikh S.: Accomodating planned exercise in Type I diabetic patients on intensive treatment. Diabetes Care 8: 337-342, 1985

Schmidt M.I., Hadji-Georgopoulos A., Rendell M., Margolis S., Kowarski D., Kowarski A.: A fasting hypoglycemia and associated free insulin and cortisol changes in "Somogyi-like" patients. Diabetes Care 2: 457–464, 1979
Schmidt M.I., Hadji-Georgopoulos A., Rendell M., Margolis S., Kowarski A.: The dawn phenomenon, an early morning glucose rise: Implications for diabetic intraday blood glucose variation. Diabetes Care 4: 579–585, 1981
Schmidt M.I., Xiong Lin Q., Gwynne J.T., Jacobs S.: Fasting early morning rise in peripheral insulin: Evidence of the dawn phenomenon in non-diabetes. Diabetes Care 7: 32–35, 1984
Schrezenmeir J., Achterberg H., Bergeler J., Küstner E., Stürmer W., Hutten H., Beyer J.: Computer-Assisted meal-related insulin therapy (CAMIT). In: Computer systems for Insulin Adjustment in Diabetes mellitus (Eds: J. Beyer, M. Albisser, J. Schrezenmeir, L. Lehmann), Proceedings of the First International Symposium on Computer Systems for Insulin Adjustment in Diabetes mellitus (Panscienta Verlag, Hedingen, Switzerland): 133-144, Mai 1987
Simpson H.C.R., Lousley S., Geekie M., Simpson R.W., Carter R.D., Hockaday T.D.R., Mann J.I.: A high carbohydrate leguminous fibre diet improves all aspects of diabetic control. Lancet 1: 1–5, 1981
Skyler J.S., Ellis G.J., Skyler D.L., Lasky I.A., Lebovitz F.L.: Insructing patients in making alterations in insulin dosage. Diabetes Care 2: 39–45, 1979
Skyler J.S., Skyler D.L., Seigler D.E., O'Sullivan M.J.: Algorithms for adjustment of insulin dosage by patients who monitor blood glucose. Diabetes Care 4: 311–318, 1981
Skyler J.S., Seigler D.E., Reeves M.L.: Optimizing pumped insulin delivery. Diabetes Care 5: 135–139, 1982
Somogyi M.: Exacerbation of diabetes by excess insulin action. Am. J. Med. 26: 169–191, 1959
Sonnenberg G.E.: Insulinpumpen. Die kontinuierliche subkutane Insulininfusion (CSII) in der Behandlung des Typ I Diabetes mellitus. Georg Thieme Verlag, Stuttgart, New York, 1983
Sonnenberg G.E., Theinert C., Hendriks M., Berger M.: Exercise and CSII: How to adjust basal and premeal insulin requirements. Diabetes 33: 69A, 1984
Teutsch S.M., Herman W.H., Dwyer D.M., Lane J.M.: Mortality among diabetic patients using continuous subcutaneous insulin infusion pumps. New Engl. J. Med. 310: 361–368, 1984
Theilgaard A., Thorsteinson B., Pinner E.M., Pramming S., Binder C.: Neuropsychological performance at different blood glucose concentrations in Type I (insulin-dependent) diabetic patients. Diabetologia 27: 338 A, 1984
Turner R.C., Phillips M., Jones R., Dornan T.L., Holman R.R.: Ultralente-based insulin regimens in insulin-dependent diabetics. In: Insulin update: 1982. (Ed.: Skyler J.S.), Exerpta Medica 157–174, Amsterdam, Genf, 1982
Vranic M., Berger M.: Exercise and diabetes mellitus. Diabetes 28: 147–163, 1979
Waldhäusl W., Bratusch-Marrain P., Gasic S., Korn A., Nowotny P.: Insulin production rate following glucose ingestion estimated by splanchic C-peptide output in normal man. Diabetologia 17: 221–227, 1979

Waldhäusl W., Bratusch-Marrain P.R., Francesconi M., Nowotny P., Kiss A.: Insulin production rate in normal man as an estimate for calibration of continuous intravenous insulin infusion in insulin dependent diabetic patients. Diabetes Care 5: 18–24, 1982

Waldhäusl W., Howorka K., Derfler K., Bratusch-Marrain P., Holler C., Zyman H., Freyler H.: Failure and efficacy of insulin therapy in insulin dependent (Type I) diabetic patients. Acta Diabetologica Latina 22: 279–294, 1985

Warram J.H., Krolewski A.S., Gottlieb M.S., Kahn C.R.: Differences in risk of insulin-dependent diabetics in offspring of diabetic mothers and diabetic fathers. New Engl. J. Med. 311: 149–152, 1984

White N.H., Skor D.A., Cryer P.E., Levandoski L.A., Bier D.M., Santiago J.V.: Identification of Type I diabetic patients at increased risk for hypoglycemia during intensive therapy. New Engl. J. Med. 308: 485–491, 1983

Wing R.R., Epstein L.H., Paternostro-Baryles M., Kriska A., Nowalk M.P., Gooding W.: Exercise in a bahavioural weight control programme for obese patients with type 2 (non-insulin-dependent) diabetes. Diabetologia 31: 902–9, 1988

Worth R., Home P.D., Johnston D.G., et al.: Intensive attention improves glycaemic control in insulin-dependent diabetes without further advantage from home blood glucose monitoring: Results of a controlled study. British Med. J. 285: 1233–1240, 1982

Appendix 1: Didactic Aspects of the FIT-Training Program

1. Prerequisites for Participation: Clarity Instead of Obscurity About the Possibilities of Therapy

It is pointless to try to force a patient to accept a complex therapeutic strategy if he does not want to try it. Provided that sufficient information is made available to him, every patient should have the opportunity to choose the form of insulin therapy that he is convinced will be best suited to his individual lifestyle and the requirements of his disease. No matter what the form of insulin therapy, since he is the one who must actually carry it out, the patient must make the final decision (see also section 4.3, "Strategies of insulin treatment"). The physician cannot do more than make his knowledge and experience available so that the decision can be made on a rational basis. Particularly for FIT, it must be remembered that the success of therapy depends on active, self-responsible execution by the patient. If the patient is not motivated, this form of therapy is simply not possible.

In order to ensure that only adequately motivated patients begin the FIT training program, it is important to explain at the very eginning (i. e., during phase 0 or 1 of rehabilitation) exactly what is involved:

- What the patient will be required to do (multiple insulin injections or insulin pump; self-monitoring of blood glucose 4-6 times per day; record-keeping and analysis, etc.).
- Advantages and disadvantages of the method as compared to other strategies of insulin therapy.

In our experience, most patients who choose conventional therapy in spite of having received comprehensive information about FIT do so, not on a rational basis, but rather – as we have seen – because they have not yet reached the stage of acceptance of the reality of their disease and have not adjusted to the changed conditions. Experience shows that many come back to the offer later, especially after hearing of the experiences of other patients.

2. Group Instead of Individual Teaching

The exchange of experiences and certain dynamic processes within groups can indeed facilitate the process of rehabilitation in chronic illness, i. e., restoration to health as far as possible ("restitutio ad optimum" instead of "restitutio ad integrum"). For this reason, the training programs during phases I and II of rehabilitation are conducted to a great extent in group form. Furthermore, since the optimal process of rehabilitation requires approximately 50 hours of training, individual teaching sessions simply would not be financially feasible. Thus, group education has the advantage of being the more efficient method as well as allowing utilization of group dynamics in order to achieve the defined learning goals.

It should be taken into consideration that with more than about 15 members in a group, clarity is lost. It is difficult, if not impossible for the leader of a large group to keep constant track of the learning process in individual members. Larger groups also require different media and methods (lecture-style) than those that are necessary for introducing intensive forms of insulin treatment.

3. Clarity Instead of Obscurity in Learning Goals

In order to have patients participate in formulating learning goals, we ask them about their wishes at the beginning of the program. A clear definition of goals also includes delineating countergoals. (Flexibility in diet should not lead to dietary chaos; self-monitoring is not the same as "constantly" having to measure blood glucose, etc.) The "Intermezzo" sections of this book represent an example of the effect of formulating countergoals.

From the standpoint of transactional analysis, the question, "What do you want out of this?" is an invitation to the Child ego state to participate in the game. In this phase of reflection the affective learning goals of the Child are combined with the cognitive goals of the Adult state when the therapist brings the patient back to reality. (You want your blood sugar to stay at 100 mg/dl forever? Do you think that's really possible?")

Participation in formulating learning goals gains in importance for the later long-term motivation of patients by helping them to identify with the contents of the training program. The better each learning goal is known and the more say patients have in determining it, the more easily they are reached and the more likely it is that the unavoidable disadvantages of the method (such as frequent blood sugar measurements and injections or pump) will be accepted as part of the bargain.

4. Working It Out for Oneself Instead of Being Presented with Material To Be Learned

A method that simply presents material to the learner (e.g., a frontal lecture) is hardly suitable for teaching a therapeutic strategy that depends on self-responsible action and adequate knowledge of the part of the patient. Such treatment strategies require continual supervision of learning by the therapist plus feedback concerning the affective and cognitive state of the learners.

Aside from offering a way of checking on the patients progress in knowledge acquisition, teaching methods which allow independent learning (teaching conversation, discussion, partner or group learning) have the advantage that patients are motivated to take part actively.

In a teaching discussion, this takes place either through

- Formulating a tentative, unsolved problem or making a paradoxical statement ("Can people who have diabetes eat foods that contain sugar? ... When would it be all right? Wouldn't there be any risks? What would you have to worry about?" ... etc.), or through
- Provocation or an attempt to anticipate a real situation that might arise ("Mrs. Meyer, imagine you have hypoglycemia and become unconscious, as has happened to you before. You land in the hospital again. After glucose infusion you regain consciousness. They want to keep you in the hospital "for observation" for a week. What do you need to consider now? What are the consequences of this event and its causes for the future? Is there anything else you can do to prevent it happening again? Will you decide to stay in the hospital as recommended? With whom would you like to talk at this particular moment? ..." etc.)

Directing a teaching conversation depends primarily on the questioning technique. The questions should be formulated in such a way that the material to be learned is worked in as answers to the questions.

The difficulty level of the questions depends on the current state of knowledge of the participants and must be adapted to the role of the individual participant in the group process, especially so that the more passive members of the group take their turn and do well, even in comparison to the most active "know-it-all." Both in teaching conversations and in less directed group discussions, the therapist should contribute in a structuring-informative manner, but should not give value judgments.

Work with a partner or in small groups are further methods that require active participation of each member. The formulation of group tasks should be clear and problem-oriented. The period of time to be taken for a specific task or solving a problem should be clearly defined and relatively brief (e.g., 15 minutes).

5. Creatively Developed Instead of Ready-Made Media

This principle arises out of teaching methods that help the learner to work things out for himself. A teaching conversation or a discussion might be structurally directed – although hardly to the degree that teaching with prestuctured media (e.g., slides) would be. The learners' knowledge and degree of participation determine the speed of the learning process and also at least part of the material taught. This material is also partly determined by the characteristics of the patients themselves and usually needs to be freshly worked out depending on the current situation. Thus, the exclusive use of prestructured media very rarely fulfills the goal of individual development of the teaching material.

Given sufficient practice, working with a blackboard or flipchart allows the simplest and most vivid development and illustration of new content and relationships. It should be remembered that the number of details in any one presentation should be kept as few as possible and that all participants should be able to read the writing.

6. No Theory or Generalisations without Concrete Examples and Immediate Consequences for Behavior

Information that is passively acquired aurally or visually is the most poorly retained. An improvement in retention can be reached by means of (a) active working out of the material by the learner (in discussions or teaching conversations) and (b) through immediate application of new material. This is the reason we decided to use as many concrete, practical exercises in insulin use as possible (fasting, "yielding to temptation," controlled raising and lowering of blood glucose etc.) If material is impossible to apply or try out immediately, imagery is used to "live through" a related situation. This is comparable to "future pace" in the model of communication and psychotherapy called neurolinguistic programming (Grinder and Bandler 1976). ("... Mr. Fox, you are planning on going skiing for two weeks in February, for a good five hours a day. What will happen to your insulin requirement? How will you recognize that? Will you be able to continue to use the rules for insulin dosage that you had been using? ..." or "Mrs. Novak, your baby is due in three months. How high should your blood sugar be during the birth? Why? What will happen to your insulin requirement when contractions begin? How will you adjust your rules for dosing insulin? ... etc.")

Appendix 2:
FIT – Initial Information for Patients

Functional, Insulin Treatment in Type I (Insulin-Dependent) Diabetes

- **Goals:**
1. Relative normoglycemia (= near-normal blood glucose levels);
2. The greatest possible freedom in dietary behavior and lifestyle.

- **Principles:**
1. Separate replacement of basal (= fasting), prandial (= meal-related) and correctional insulin;
2. Self-monitoring of blood glucose as a substitute for continuous blood glucose (blood sugar) measurement by the pancreas.

- **Methods:**
1. Insulin replacement (= insulin substitution) by means of multiple injections or a programmable insulin infusion pump;
2. Self-monitoring of blood sugar about 4 times a day;
3. Immediate correction of blood sugar when it is off-target.

The release of insulin, and thus the control of metabolism is governed by a number of mechanisms in the healthy body. The purpose of this fine regulation is to ensure that the amount of insulin in the blood is adjusted to need, depending on the concentration of nutrients such as glucose or protein at any given time.

In a healthy body, the pancreas produces an average of about one unit (U) of insulin every hour if nothing is eaten, i. e., under basal conditions. That would be about 24 U per day. This basal insulin serves to maintain normal blood glucose levels of about 100 mg/dl in a fasting condition. When food is consumed, the healthy pancreas releases on the average an additional 1.4 units of insulin per unit of carbohydrates (one carbohydrate unit = 12 g carbohydrates = 50 calories) and 0.5

units of insulin per 100 calories of protein and fat. These figures approximately represent the insulin need of a type I (insulin-dependent) diabetic person with a usual insulin need of about 40 to 50 units per day.

With a normal diet, less than half of the insulin released by the pancreas is secreted under fasting conditions (basal insulin), and the rest is produced in order to compensate for food intake (prandial insulin).

The amount of insulin needed each day varies from person to person, depending on slight differences in the insulin sensitivity of the body and on body weight. Puberty, pregnancy, fever, severe fluid loss, serious injuries, stress and medications (for example, some birth control pills) can all cause reductions in insulin sensitivity. (When body cells become less sensitive to insulin, more insulin would be needed to do the same job.) Kidney disease or some conditions where there is a deficiency of a certain hormone can cause body cells to become relatively oversensitive to insulin. (The more sensitive the body cells are to insulin, the less insulin is needed.) Physical activity (sport) can also reduce insulin requirement.

Insulin-Dependent Diabetes and Its Treatment

If there is not enough insulin in the body, it must be replaced. Since the discovery of insulin in 1922, this replacement has been carried out by injecting a prescribed amount of insulin and keeping to a rigid diet (= "conventional insulin therapy"). This type of therapy, which was determined by the doctor, was able to prevent severe metabolic derangement and decisively prolong the patient's life. It meant, however, that food intake and insulin injections had to be carried out at predetermined times and that the amount and type of food were determined by the blood sugar-lowering effect of the insulin injected. This situation forced patients to live a strictly regimented life.

Functional Insulin Treatment (FIT)

In contrast to conventional insulin treatment, FIT is based on the separation of the insulin needed in a fasting condition (= basal insulin) from the insulin needed to compensate for food intake (= prandial insulin) and from the insulin needed for correction of high blood sugar. This procedure imitates insulin production in a healthy person and allows a responsible, trained diabetic person to achieve good metabolic control while maintaining a flexible life-style.

Achieving the (realizable!) goal of combining flexibility and good metabolic control does require proper training and continual participation on the part of the patient. It is necessary to take part in a training program in order to learn how to choose the correct insulin for any given meal, whether in everyday life or in special situations.

The important building blocks for successful, near-normoglycemic, functional insulin treatment (FIT) are made up of thorough knowledge of and ability to carry out the following:

- Compositon of food (carbohydrates, protein, fat, energy content);
- Rules for insulin dosage – the algorithms for FIT;
- Basal insulin;
- Prandial insulin;
- Self-monitoring and use of insulin for correction;
- Keeping a self-monitoring diary.

Composition of Food

Only exact knowledge of the nature of each food you eat allows you to determine how much prandial insulin you need. In the learning phase, it is absolutely necessary to use a diet scale.

Rules for Insulin Dosage – the Algorithms for FIT

Initial guidelines for insulin dosage (algorithms) for most patients with a daily insulin requirement of about 40-50 U would be:

Basal insulin (U/24 h):	approx. 20 U
Prandial insulin:	1.3 U per carbohydrate unit (12 g CHO)
	0.5 U per 100 kcal of protein/fat

The insulin for protein/fat is only needed for meals that are low in carbohydrates. These values need to individually adjusted, since insulin sensitivity varies from person to person.

Basal Insulin

You can replace basal insulin either with an insulin infusion pump or by subcutaneously injecting approximately equal amounts of a delayed-acting insulin. To compensate for the decrease in insulin sensitivity (increased insulin requirement) that usually occurs in the morning, you can inject a small amount of fast-acting regular insulin (2-6 U) as a part of the basal dose. As example of basal insulin dosage for a patient with a total daily insulin requirement of 40-50 U would be as follows:

Morning dose:	12 U delayed-acting insulin
	3 U regular insulin
Evening dose:	12 U delayed-acting insulin

You can assume that your basal insulin dose is right for you if:

1. *Your blood sugar remains stable between meals and overnight;*
2. *Your fasting blood sugar values are at or near your target level (usually between 90 and 140 mg/dl); and*
3. *The amount of delayed-acting insulin you inject is not more than half of your total daily insulin dose.*

If this is not the case, you should adapt your insulin dose accordingly. Sometimes, especially if you often have fasting values that are too high, it may be advisable to change the type of insulin you inject at bedtime to one which would have its peak action in the early morning (for example, an NPH or lente insulin).

Prandial Insulin

You should use only fast-acting regular insulin to fulfill your prandial (food-related) insulin needs. It should not be mixed with delayed-acting insulins in the same syringe. The amount of insulin you need to cover the food you eat depends mainly on the following factors:

- Amount of carbohydrates;
- Type of carbohydrates and how they were processed (whether finely ground, well-cooked, etc.);
- Protein and fat content of the meal;
- Fiber content;
- Whether and how much liquid you drink with the meal.
- The time during the day, when you eat.

You can assume that the dosage you used for a particular meal was correct if your blood sugar is neither too high nor too low several hours (about 4 h) after eating **(late postprandial values)**. This will mean that the amount of carbohydrates you ate was balanced by the proper amount of insulin. **Early postprandial values** (one to two hours after eating) tell you more about the t iming of the carbohydrate and/or insulin absorption into your bloodstream. Especially when you eat a large meal, you can speed up the absorption of the insulin into your bloodstream by injecting into the muscle rather than just under the skin, for example by injecting into your lower arm. You can also speed up insulin absorption from the fatty tissue under your skin by massaging the place where you inject.

Blood Glucose Correction

Your goal will usually be to achieve the following blood sugar levels:

For fasting and before meals:	about 100 mg/dl
After a meal (= postprandially):	1 h below 160 mg/d l
	2 h below 140 mg/dl

These target levels may have to be modified if, for example, you have a history of severe hypoglycemia (then you would choose slightly higher target levels), or if you are pregnant (then you would choose slightly lower target levels).

If you test your blood sugar and find that it is off-target, then a blood glucose correction is necessary; either injecting regular insulin to lower a blood sugar value that is too high, or consuming glucose to raise a value that is too low. In deciding on a correction, you will have to consider the interval since your last correction of a value that was too high. You should wait at least 3 hours since your last correction before making another correction. (But you can correct anytime after a prandial injection if you find that your blood sugar is high.) Here is an example of the guidelines (algorithms) for estimating how much insulin or glucose is necessary for correction in a patient whose insulin requirement is about average:

- Change in blood sugar produced by 1 U regular insulin: −40 mg/dl
- Change in blood sugar produced by 1 carbohydrate unit: +50 mg/dl (12 g carbohydrates)

Self-Monitoring

The insulin-producing cells of a healthy pancreas continually measure blood glucose and release their insulin accordingly. Self-monitoring and correcting your blood sugar is an attempt to imitate this control function. Of course, you won't do it as often as the cells of a pancreas would, but you will need to test your blood sugar 4 or 5 times a day in order to dose your insulin correctly if you wish to achieve near-normal HbA_{1c} values. (HbA_{1c} is the laboratory value that tells you approximately what your average blood sugar has been for at least the last few weeks.) In the training program you will learn how to use both blood glucose test strips that can be evaluated directly on the basis of color and strips that are inserted into a glucose meter. The most important time points for measuring blood sugar are:

1. Late in the evening, at bedtime;
2. When you wake up (fasting);
3. Spot tests before and/or after eating;
4. Whenever you suspect that you might be hypoglycemic.

Urine glucose tests can only tell you whether your blood sugar has gone above your kidney threshold for glucose. For this reason it is better to use blood glucose tests as a basis for decisions about insulin dosage.

Acetone (ketones) in your urine (also measured with test strips) tells you either that you do not have enough insulin in your bloodstream (if blood sugar is also high and/or there is sugar in your urine) or that you are not eating enough (if blood sugar is normal).

Keeping a Self-Monitoring Diary

It is important to keep a daily record of the following:

Insulin (type and amount)
Blood sugar (mg/dl)
Food intake (number of carbohydrate units; 1 unit = 12 g)
Problems (for example, hypoglycemia, illness, etc.)

▷

Fig. A 2.1. Profile of insulin action (1) and glucose in serum (2) in healthy persons. Insulin action under FIT is represented in (3).

Pump or multiple injections . . .

. . . the patient decides!

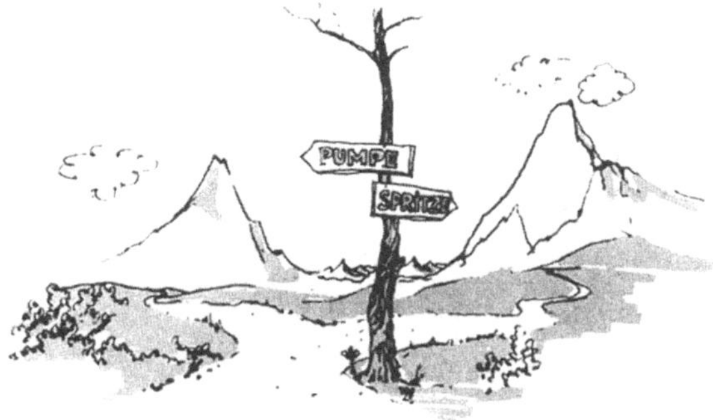

DAILY PROFILE of INSULIN ACTION and BLOOD GLUCOSE in HEALTHY PERSONS

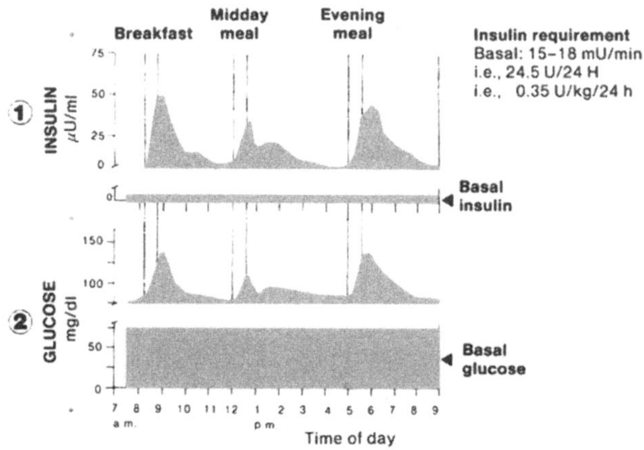

Schematic representation of insulin action under FIT

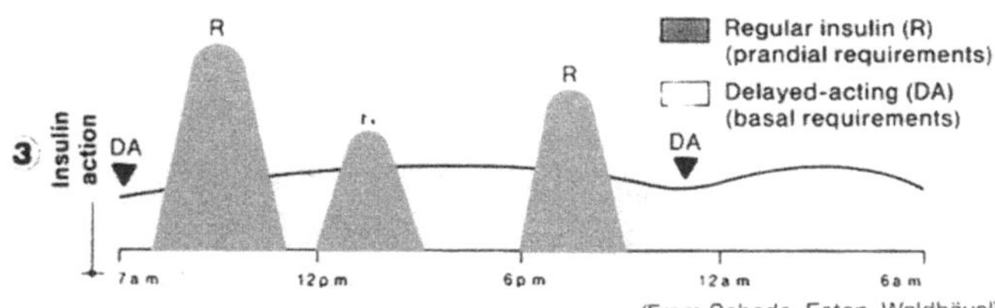

(From Schade, Eaton, Waldhäusl)

To make decisions on insulin dosage properly, you will need to make a daily "accounting" of mean blood glucose, total amount of regular insulin and delayed-acting insulin and total food intake. The net result of this analysis gives you a basis for modifying your individual guidelines for insulin dosage (algorithms) and serves as a basis for consultations with your doctor and/or diabetes counselor.

Summary

Functional, near-normoglycemic insulin treatment (FIT) requires:

- Acquiring the necessary knowledge through a training program in FIT;
- Separate administration of delayed-acting and regular insulin or use of a programmable insulin infusion pump.
- Replacement of prandial insulin before each meal.
- Self-monitoring of blood sugar at least 4 times a day, if you wish to achieve near-normal HbA_{1c} levels.
- Immediate correction of blood glucose values that deviate from your target level (fasting: 100 mg/dl; after meals: 160 mg/dl).
- Autonomous modification of algorithms for insulin dosage if there is a change in insulin requirement.
- Keeping a self-monitoring diary and using it as a basis for consultation with the diabetes center.

Functional, near-normoglycemic insulin treatment (FIT) allows:

- Good metabolic control with relative freedom from hypoglycemia;
- The greatest possible adjustment of therapy to your lifestyle and individual circumstances.

Appendix 3: Nomogramm for Generating the Initial Algorithms for FIT

Coauthors: H. Egger and H. Thoma

The tables presented here were devised on the basis of statistical analysis of data from 158 FIT patients. The baseline data from each patient – weight, height, HbA_{1c}, ketonuria, urine glucose, mean blood glucose (MBG), daily insulin requirement, diet (carbohydrate units per day) – were determined within the first three days of the hospital stay before the beginning of the FIT program (i. e., under conventional or intensified therapy). They were then related to the individually "optimized" algorithms from the end of the training program (MBG 118 $\pm$21) by means of stepwise regression in order to generate the nomogram (Egger 1986). For simplification, the baseline data were reduced to the two statistically most relevant parameters, the total daily insulin dose (U/day) and the daily mean blood glucose value (10-12 values per day, including postprandial values). The original calculation of the initial algorithms for FIT was based on all of the parameters mentioned above and is available on an IBM-compatible disk.

The basal delayed-acting insulin is divided into two approximately equal portions and administered twice daily. When NPH or lente insulins are used for the basal dose, the evening dose should be administered late, just before going to bed, never before the evening meal. For "combined" basal insulinization with ultralente in the morning and NPH or lente at bedtime, and for CSII, the total basal dose (per 24 h) given in the nomogram should be reduced by approx. 10–5%. The algorithms for basal and prandial insulin are given in IU, while the blood glucose values in the algorithms for correction are given in mg/dl.

Abbreviations: MBG = mean blood glucose (mg/dl)
Insulin = mean daily insulin requirement (IU/24 h)

MBG	100	120	140	160	180	200	220	240	260	280	300
Insulin											
10	3	4	5	6	6	7	8	9	10	10	11
14	5	6	7	8	9	9	10	11	12	13	14
18	7	8	8	9	10	11	12	13	13	14	15
22	8	9	10	11	12	13	13	14	15	16	17
26	10	11	11	12	13	14	15	16	17	18	19
30	11	12	13	14	15	16	16	17	18	19	20
34	12	13	14	15	16	17	18	19	20	21	22
38	14	15	16	16	17	18	19	20	21	22	23
42	15	16	17	18	19	20	21	21	22	23	24
46	16	17	18	19	20	21	22	23	24	25	26
50	18	19	20	21	22	23	24	25	26	27	28
54	19	20	21	22	23	24	25	26	27	28	29
58	20	21	22	23	24	25	26	27	28	30	31
62	21	22	23	24	26	27	28	29	30	31	32
66	23	24	25	26	27	28	29	30	31	32	33
* 70	24	25	26	27	28	29	30	31	32	33	34
* 74	25	26	27	28	29	30	31	32	33	35	36
* 78	26	27	28	29	30	31	33	34	35	36	37
* 82	27	28	30	31	32	33	34	35	36	37	38
* 86	29	30	31	32	33	34	35	36	37	38	39
* 90	30	31	32	33	34	35	36	37	38	39	40
* 94	31	32	33	34	35	36	37	38	40	41	42

Fig. A 3.1a.* Amount of basal long-acting insulin per day.

MBG	100	150	200	250	300
Insulin					
10	2	2	3	3	3
20	2	3	3	3	4
30	3	3	3	4	4
40	3	4	4	4	5
50	4	4	4	5	5
60	4	5	5	5	6
70*	5	5	5	5	6
80*	6	5	6	6	7
90*	6	7	6	7	9
100*	6	7	7	9	10

Fig. A 3.1b. Component of regular insulin in the morning basal dose.

* With high daily insulin requirements it is advisable to use also an evening regular insulin as an integrated basal component to keep the dose for delayed acting insulin a low as possible.

MBG:	100	120	140	160	180	200	220	240	260	280	300
Insulin											
10	0,4	0,5	0,6	0,6	0,7	0,8	0,8	0,9	1.0	1.0	1,1
14	0,5	0,5	0,6	0,7	0,7	0,8	0,9	0,9	1.0	1,1	1,2
18	0,5	0,6	0,7	0,7	0,8	0,9	0,9	1.0	1,1	1,1	1,2
22	0,6	0,7	0,7	0,8	0,9	0,9	1.0	1,1	1,1	1,2	1,3
26	0,7	0,7	0,8	0,9	0,9	1.0	1,1	1,2	1,2	1,3	1,4
30	0,8	0,8	0,9	1.0	1.0	1,1	1,2	1,2	1,3	1,4	1,4
34	0,9	0,9	1.0	1,1	1,1	1,2	1,3	1,4	1,4	1,5	1,6
38	1.0	1,1	1,1	1,2	1,3	1,3	1,4	1,5	1,5	1,6	1,7
42	1,1	1,2	1,3	1,3	1,4	1,5	1,5	1,6	1,7	1,7	1,8
46	1,3	1,3	1,4	1,5	1,6	1,6	1,7	1,8	1,8	1,9	2.0
50	1,4	1,5	1,6	1,6	1,7	1,8	1,8	1,9	2.0	2,1	2,1
54	1,6	1,7	1,8	1,8	1,9	2.0	2.0	2,1	2,2	2,2	2,3
58	1,8	1,9	1,9	2.0	2,1	2,1	2,2	2,3	2,3	2,4	2,5
62	2.0	2,1	2,1	2,2	2,3	2,3	2,4	2,5	2,5	2.6	2,7
66	2,2	2,3	2,4	2,4	2,5	2,6	2,6	2,7	2,8	2,8	2,9
70	2,4	2,5	2,6	2,7	2,7	2,8	2,9	2,9	3.0	3,1	3,1
74	2,7	2,8	2,8	2,9	3.0	3.0	3,1	3,2	3,2	3,3	3,4
78	2,9	3.0	3,1	3,2	3,2	3,3	3,4	3,4	3,5	3,6	3,6
82	3.0	3,1	3,2	3,3	3,4	3,5	3,6	3,7	3,8	3,9	4.0
86	3,2	3,3	3,4	3,5	3,6	3,7	3,8	3,9	4.0	4,1	4,2
90	3,5	3,6	3,7	3,8	3,9	4.0	4,1	4,2	4,3	4,4	4,5
94	3,7	3,8	3,9	4.0	4,1	4,3	4,4	4,5	4,6	4,7	4,8
98	4.0	4,1	4,2	4,3	4,4	4,5	4,6	4,7	4,8	4,9	5.0

Fig. A 3.1c. Amount of prandial (regular) insulin per carbohydrate unit (12 g CHO).

MBG	100	150	200	250	300
Insulin					
10	0.1	0.2	0.2	0.3	0.3
20	0.2	0.3	0.3	0.4	0.4
30	0.3	0.4	0.4	0.5	0.5
40	0.4	0.5	0.5	0.6	0.6
50	0.5	0.5	0.6	0.6	0.7
60	0.6	0.6	0.7	0.7	0.8
70	0.7	0.7	0.8	0.8	0.9
80	0.8	0.8	0.9	0.9	1,0
90	0.9	0.9	1,0	1,0	1,0
100	0.9	1,0	1,0	1,0	1,0

Fig. A 3.1d. Amount of prandial (regular) insulin per 100 kcal of protein/fat. Insulin substitution for protein/fat is necessary only for meals that are low in carbohydrates.

MBG	100	150	200	250	300
Insulin					
10	90	85	80	70	65
20	85	75	65	60	60
30	70	60	55	55	55
40	60	55	50	50	45
50	45	45	40	40	40
60	40	35	35	35	30
70	35	30	30	30	25
80	30	30	25	20	20
90	25	20	15	15	10

Fig. A 3.1e. Delta BG: Amount that blood glucose is lowered by 1 U of regular insulin. This value should be increased (i.e., a greater drop should be assumed) in situations that have a h igh risk of hypoglycemia (for example, at the beginning of FIT) and for patients with characteristics that increase the risk of severe hypoglycemia.

Weight	45	50	55	60	65	70	75	80	85	90	95
Delta BG	60	55	50	50	50	45	45	45	40	40	35

Fig. A 3.1f. Delta BG: Amount that blood glucose is raised by 1 carbohydrate unit (12 g CHO = 50 kcal from carbohydrates).

Appendix 4: Selection of Available Human Insulins*

Most insulin manufacturers currently produce all of the insulin types mentioned here (regular, NPH/isophane, lente, ultralente).

* A large number of mixtures of regular and delayed-acting insulins in varying proportions are commercially available. Since these premixed insulins are not suitable for the purposes of FIT, they are not listed here.

** According to Bottermann et al. 1985 (in dosage of 0.3 IU per kg body weight; activity profiles as examples for insulins of NOVO-NORDISK). With the small amounts of insulin per dose resulting from the separate administration of basal, prandial and correctional insulin required by FIT, the duration of activity can be expected to be correspondingly shorter.

*** The insulin analog Lispro (Humalog®, ELI LILLY) has a considerably faster effect than regular insulin. The activity curve shown here is based on an insulin dosage of 10 units (i.e., less than half the dosage shown in the examples of other insulin types; Galloway 1993).

Insulin type (delaying substance)	Pharmacokinetics** (Examples)	Manufacturer		
		HOECHST	LILLY	NOVO-NORDISK
Rapid acting analog Regular insulin	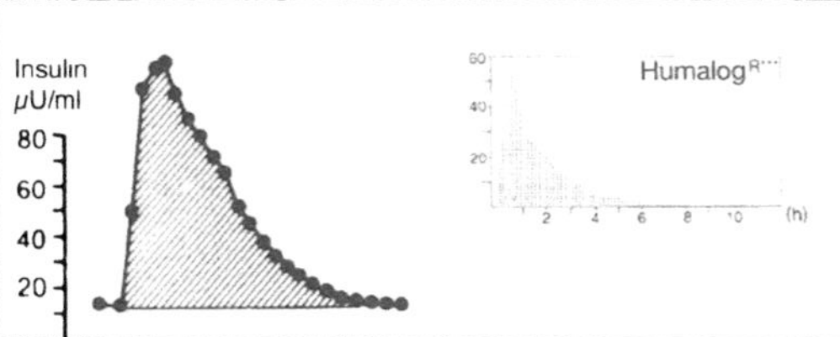	Insuman Rapid	(Insulin-analog Lispro) Humalog^R Humulin R	Novalin R
NPH (Protamine)	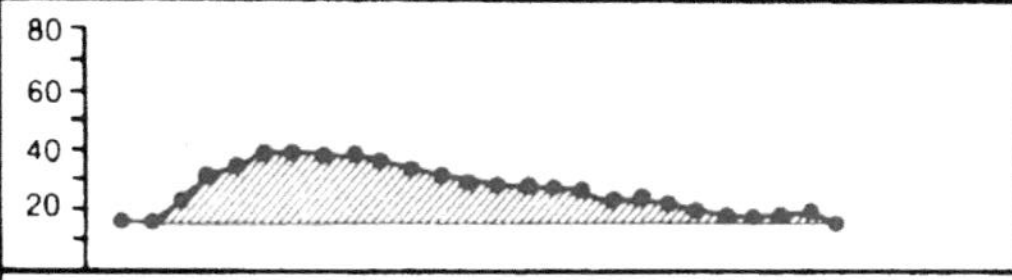	Insuman Basal	Humulin N	Novalin N
Lente (Zinc amorphous + crystalline)	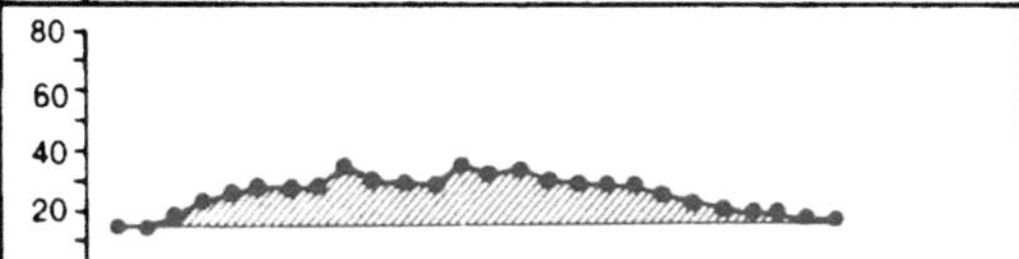		Humulin L	Novalin L
Ultralente (crystalline)	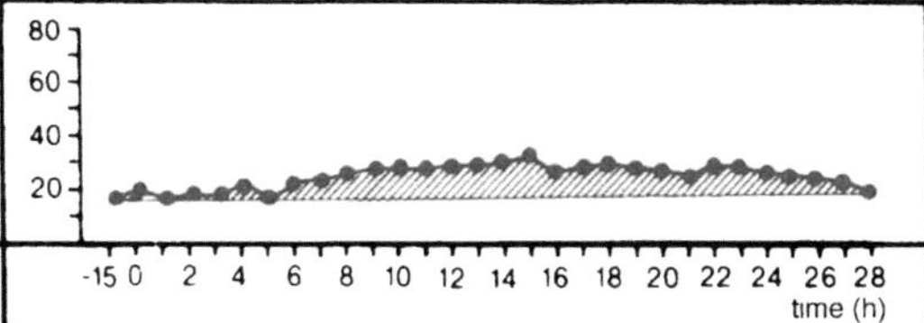		Humulin U	Novalin U

Appendix 5: Examples of Carbohydrate Units

One CHO Unit = 12 g carbohydrates (50 kcal from carbohydrates).

Foods are listed in amounts containing 1 CHO unit. Those products which contain protein and/or fat also contain correspondingly more calories.

Bread and Cereals		
Wholemeal bread	25 g	1 small slice
White bread	20 g	1/2 thick slice
Roll	20 g	1/2 large roll
Crispbread, rye crisp	15 g	as indicated on package
Pasta	15 g	uncooked, 1 tablespoon
	50 g	cooked, 2–3 tablespoons
Rice	15 g	uncooked, 1 level tablespoon
	50 g	cooked, 2 level tablespoons
Flour	15 g	1 level tablespoon
Vegetables		
Potatoes	60 g	1 egg-sized potato boiled or roast
Lentils	20 g	uncooked, 2 tablespoons
	55 g	cooked
Beans, peas, dried	20 g	uncooked, 2 tablespoons
	55 g	cooked
Sweet corn	60 g	cooked, 5 tablespoons
Fruit		
Apple	100 g	1 small
Orange	130 g	1 medium, without skin
Peach	120 g	1 medium

Banana	60 g	1/2 medium, without skin
Pineapple	100 g	1 slice
Fruitjuice (orange, pineapple)	125 g	1 small glass (4 oz.)

Milk Products

Milk, whole or skimmed	250 g	1 cup (approx. 8 oz.)
Joghurt	250 g	1 cup (approx. 8 oz.)

Subject Index

(**Boldface** page numbers refer to the most comprehensive descriptions. ff. = and following pages)

Springer-Verlag and the Environment

We at Springer-Verlag firmly believe that an international science publisher has a special obligation to the environment, and our corporate policies consistently reflect this conviction.

We also expect our business partners – paper mills, printers, packaging manufacturers, etc. – to commit themselves to using environmentally friendly materials and production processes.

The paper in this book is made from low- or no-chlorine pulp and is acid free, in conformance with international standards for paper permanency.

MIX
Papier aus verantwortungsvollen Quellen
Paper from responsible sources
FSC® C105338

If you have any concerns about our products,
you can contact us on
ProductSafety@springernature.com

In case Publisher is established outside the EU,
the EU authorized representative is:
Springer Nature Customer Service Center GmbH
Europaplatz 3, 69115 Heidelberg, Germany

Printed by Libri Plureos GmbH
in Hamburg, Germany